Introducing Psychology

How To Analyze People With Cognitive Psychology. Positive Personality Coaching Series. A Behavioral Psychological Mastery Approach. Create New Habits To Support Your Mindset

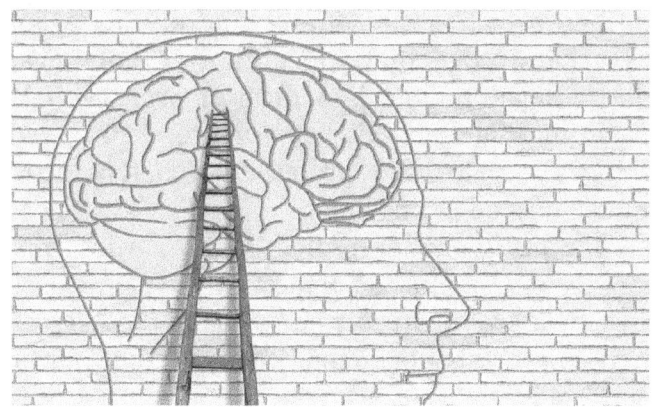

By DR. Felicity Gray

Contents

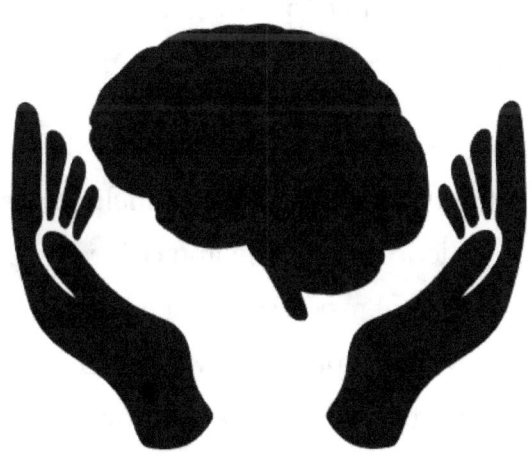

Introduction

Psychology mainly deals with studying the conscious and unconscious occurrences. In turn, Psychologists study the thoughts and feelings of people. They aim is to understand how the brain functions, and its role in shaping the behavior people. They all work towards the understanding of how people make decisions, and the reasons for doing so.

It is through psychology that one is able to understand, explain and describe why people behave as they do, as well as the reasons behind them. People are able to understand human behavior through analysis, identifying the behavior and describing the reasons why it has been developed. After that, the psychologists are able to determine its cause, and how the behavior can be controlled.

Psychology has determining factors that enable people to understand it better. Those factors include explaining, describing, prediction, changing and controlling people's behaviors and mental processes. Psychologists must take their time when studying people's behavior. This is because they have to ensure that they get all details concerning the person's behavior, without error, in order to correct the behavior. If it is bad behavior, they should be able to correct it early enough and good behavior nurtured.

There are so many psychologists out there who are experienced in different fields of psychology. Their aim is to make sure that people have meaningful relationships with the people around them, and that their behavior is positive. Psychologists make sure that they correct the bad behavior, by instilling good behavior. They can do this through rewards or punishments.

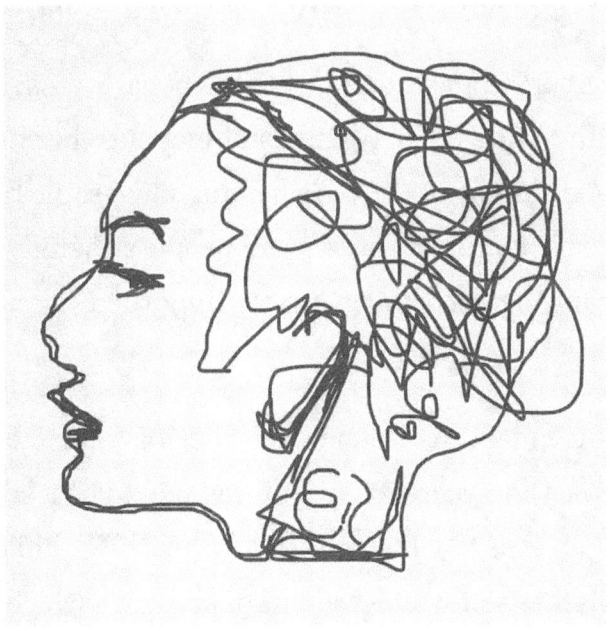

Chapter 1: Psychology Definition

What Is Psychology?

Psychology is referred to as the study of people's behavior, as well as their minds. Psychology can also be defined as the process of applying the knowledge which enables people to understand events, to ensure that their mental health is good, to improve people's education levels, improve their relationships among themselves and in a working environment.

Apart from studying people's behavior, psychology deals with a wide range of things. It includes the study of human development, people's health, how people behave socially, sports, clinical issues and people's cognitive processes. This means that psychology is very important in our everyday lives.

As much as it is a new science, it is said to have evolved over the last 150 years. Its origin was said to be traced back to Ancient Greece, which was 400- 500 years BC. Philosophers would discuss some topics about psychology, which they were familiar with. They would discuss nature and how it was affecting them, as well as determinism and attractions. Those are the topics that they would mostly discuss and relate them to their way of living. Later on, psychology became a discipline. Theories were developed to discuss how the brain worked, its structure and how it functions.

What Does Psychology Include?

Psychology is very important in people's lives. After all, once one has knowledge about psychology, they are able to gain insight into the reasons why they behave in a certain way. They are also able to understand the people around them, since they understand their behavior and reasons for behaving the way they do. This makes them able to interact well with people around them as they understand their actions.

The psychologists learn all people's behavior, how their behavior impacts their lives and how it relates to the pressures in society. Psychologists apply everything they learn to the treatment of mental cases, enhancing people's behavior whether negative or positive, and also in self-help. Furthermore, it is applied in many other areas, related to health in people's day-to-day lives.

The psychologists are also said to research human development, their personality, as well as thoughts, feelings, and emotions; including the things that motivate people and their social behavior. Psychology is so broad, considering it touches almost all areas of human life. There have been many misconceptions about psychology. This may have resulted from its many branches that are understood by people differently.

You will find that there are those psychologists who help people in dealing with crimes, while there are others who deal with only mental issues. Also, psychologists may ensure that people have workplaces with a good work environment. We can, therefore, agree that different psychologists perform different tasks, but their goals are equal. Their main objective is to make sure that they describe situations, predict the outcomes and give an explanation for their findings. They then relate all their findings to human behavior, and how each of their finds relates to how people behave.

What Are The Goals Of Psychology?

Although many may understand how psychology works, there are also plenty other people who do not understand it. They may not be aware of its goals, and why it is necessary. It would be therefore detrimental to explain the goals of psychology, for it to be understood by everyone. Below are the goals of psychology.

Describe

The first objective of psychology is said to be describing someone's behavior. It is through the description of the behaviors in both people and animals, in which a better understanding is gained. When they are understood, they are able to handle them, depending on their behavior. This helps a lot in avoiding conflicts when interacting with them, and also when at work. With a good understanding of psychology, one is also able to understand what behaviors are normal, and those that are not. When someone describes to you how they feel, you fit in their shoes and try to imagine that feeling, becoming empathetic. This enables you to be able to help them out of the situations facing them. This is exactly how psychologists are able to describe the behavior of the people they interacted with.

Psychological researchers are said to use many research tools in order for them to describe behavior. They may use naturalistic observation, which is described as using the objects you would want to research on, when they are in their natural environment. The naturalistic observations are carried out in an area where the research cannot in a laboratory. This helps psychologists observe the behaviors, as they happen. By doing this, they can obtain a better understanding, as they see people's reactions, while they are happening to them.

Another tool that is used by psychologists is the correlational studies that involve looking at a relationship between two, or even more variables. By looking at the relationship, one will be able to tell if the relationship exists or not. However, correlational studies are not in a position to tell why the relationship between the two variables is not working, or why it is working. This means that a researcher should be in a position to identify the best time to use this method, in a particular situation. This will help in ensuring that the researcher gets the most appropriate results in their study.

The researchers also use self-report inventories in their research. This method is mostly used for the assessment of one's personality. It is of great help, because it helps people answer questions about various things in life. They are able to write down their strengths and weaknesses, which help them find out where they are failing, in life. The self-report inventories test enables them to work on their weaknesses. The researchers may also use case studies and surveys to describe people's behavior.

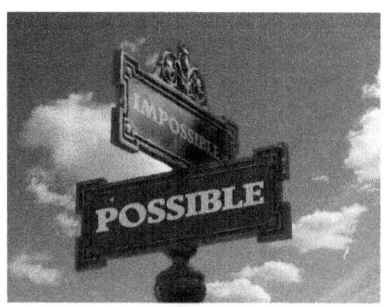

To Explain

The second goal of explaining people's behavior is to explain. It involves giving an explanation of the reasons for people's behavior. It is through the explanations that people are able to understand the situations facing them, and how they can be helped. There are so many people who have come up with theories to explain human behavior. One of the theories, being classical conditioning, mainly talks about behaviorism. Behaviorism states that we all learn by interacting with the environment. It is through the environment that we acquire some behaviors. It also states that the environment shapes how people behave. It theorizes that people may have earlier on acquired good behavior, but when they interact with people with bad behavior, they automatically acquire bad behavior. The environment you are in therefore, dictates how you will behave. In order to ensure that people nurture good behavior, it would be important to ensure that they stay in an environment, that is filled with positivity.

There is also the Attachment Theory, which focusses on people's relationships, and whether their bonds are good or not. The bond may be between the parents and their children, or even two people who may be courting. Through the theory, one is able to analyze and give reasons why the bond between two people is strong or weak.

To Control

After we learn the reasons why people behave the way they do, we would want to have some control over it in the future. We can only do this by coming up with ways of preventing a repeat of some situations in the future. For example, when we observe and predict that you might choose a partner who is abusive, just because your parents were abusive, we can make sure that you do not choose that partner. People can be sent to talk to you and give you an insight into why you would be advised to think through your choice, before committing yourself to it. This will help in ensuring that the cycle does not repeat. By doing this, you will have taken control of the situation. As a human being, being in control of the environment that we are in is very important. This will help us to be able to protect ourselves from negativity, and also work on our weaknesses. We will also be able to help the people around us have control over their behavior.

To Predict

This goal is used to predict the reasons for certain behavior. It normally predicts how people think and act, as well as reasons why they think and act that way. Through the predictions, it is possible to assume the outcome of a certain behavior, even before it happens. One can also be able to predict the next time that the behavior is likely to happen, why it will happen and how it might happen. Through the predictions, one can prevent certain outcomes. Another one will be able to come up with measures that will help ensure that bad behavior is not repeated.

Predicting behavior has also been helpful to people since they are able to understand a lot of underlying issues that they would not understand in the past. This enables them to understand the reasons why people act the way they do. The psychologists are also able to make correct guesses about human behavior, without too much effort.

To Change

The last goal is to change. Most psychologists aim to make changes about some behaviors, and to influence and control one's behavior, which would in return, enable people to experience a positive change in their behavior. They study human behavior, analyze it and come up with ways of changing the bad behavior, improving the good one. By doing this, people are able to experience positive change in their lives, which motivates them to do even better in the future.

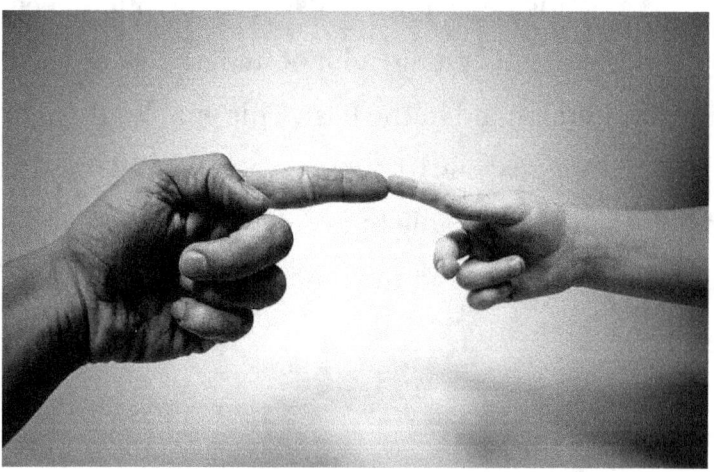

Is Psychology Important In Our Everyday Lives?

Psychology is very important in our daily lives. This is because psychologists study people's behavior as well as their mental state. People's behavior and mental state are crucial in their day-to-day lives. In short, it helps people interact well with people. They are able to understand each other, even as they carry out their daily activities.

Psychology is also important since it enables people to understand the reasons for people's behavior. People are able to understand people's actions, the reasons for the decisions they make and also how they think. It is easy to understand reasons why people stop their previous behavior and start behaving differently.

Through psychology, one is able to predict people's behavior and control the behavior that is not pleasant. By doing this, people will change their reactions to situations, by applying better conflict resolution strategies. People are also able to shape their behavior through psychology. Those with negative behavior are able to correct their behavior little by little in order for them to acquire better behaviors. They are able to evaluate themselves with the help of a psychologist, and be able to come up with better ways to accomplish tasks, and offer better approaches to conflicts. By doing this, people are able to relate well with others. They are also able to accommodate people with their flaws, and work well with them without experiencing any challenges.

For those with positive behavior, they are able to improve it to become even better. They can help those experiencing challenges with their behavior to acquire good behavior. They will be influencing them positively, which helps to make them live a positivity filled life.

Psychology is also used in the study of some diseases, such as Alzheimer's and Parkinson's disease. The psychologists are able to study the diseases and come up with the way in which they can help the patients manage the diseases. They have also been able to find a cure for some of these diseases, which have been of great help to the patients, since they are able to live comfortably with the medication. The psychologists are also able to guide and counsel the caregivers of these patients, in order for them to comfortably take care of these patients without getting too emotionally drained.

Another benefit of psychology is that we are able to understand ourselves. We can be able to give reasons why we may be behaving the way we do, and how to overcome the behavior. We are also able to learn more about our personality, our weaknesses, and even our strengths. When people understand themselves, they are able to come up with goals that they would want to achieve, and make sure that they achieve them. This is because they have the motivation required to achieve their goals. They also take everything seriously, because they know what it means to be able to achieve the set goals.

Another benefit of psychology is enabling people to have self-confidence. When people learn and understand their personality, they are able to become more confident in themselves. This is because they know how to deal with all their weaknesses. Self-confidence is of great importance in one's life, because you cannot be shaken by any challenges when you believe in yourself.

One's self-esteem also improves when one has confidence. They are able to feel good about themselves; with little steps they are able to see progress in their lives.

There are so many people who have studied psychology as a career. Studying is one's personal choice so no one can be forced to study it. There are many reasons why someone would choose to study psychology. Some of the reasons have been discussed below.

Learn Reasons Why People Act Weirdly

There are many reasons why people act strangely. It would be idealistic to discover some of those reasons. This is one reason enough to choose psychology instead of any other subject. In a chapter like social psychology, you will be able to understand why certain people would rush to help, while others wouldn't move a muscle to help. Your curiosity will enable you to want to discover why people behave differently. Studying psychology is all fun as you learn the behavior of others, because you will also be able to study your behavior. Is there anything more fun than that?

You Learn How to Do Thorough Research

When one joins a university or a college, you get various skills. One of them is doing research in this field. It is through research that one is able to discover various things about psychology. One will be engaged in so many researches that you will start thinking critically about all issues. The research will be helpful in ensuring that one gets the skills required to handle issues related to this field. As they do their research, they are able to gain a lot of knowledge and skills in ways of handling different issues. This will be of great help in ensuring that you will be of help to people with psychological issues, once you are through with your studies. Through research, a psychology student will be able to learn about the important research tools, which they can use when handling people.

To Learn About the Different Mental Disorders and the Available Treatment Options

There are many psychologists who battle with psychological disorders. They may not even be aware of the treatment options available for them to treat their disorders. This means that as they do research about the treatments, they will also be able to get their own treatment. They will have killed two birds with one stone. They will be able to help other people who may be encountering similar problems, and they will also get help in the process.

To Get Insight into People's Behavior

Through psychology, a student will be able to study all forms of human behavior. This means that you will learn the differences in human behavior, as well as all the characteristics of human behavior. The psychology student will, therefore, be able to get answers to everything related to human behavior. As they learn that, they will also be able to discover some of their behaviors that are pleasant, and those that are not. Through the insights, they will be able to help people with these issues, because they have already experienced them first hand. They also are able to understand people's behavior and the reasons for that behavior.

It is therefore important for people to consider studying psychology as a career, as this will help them learn many things related to people's behavior, and their mental state which will in return help them, help people to live a healthy life; one that is filled with positive traits. Psychology is also said to be one of the most highly paid jobs. We all want a career that can cater for all our bills. Why not study psychology?

What is the Perspective of Psychology?

I am sure at one point you have questioned yourself on the reasons for behaving the way you do. You will find yourself remembering certain things, and not remembering some. You will also find out that some people prefer staying indoors, while others would rather go out all night. Someone who has studied psychology will easily understand all the above. This is because most of them have studied the mind, as well as how it works, and even how it was used in the past. The aspects of human behavior have been studied in the before, of course. The psychologists studied how the brain functions, people's personality and also the influences that are brought about by how people relate to each other.

It is clear that structuralism has already been replacing the approach of psychology. The approaches have been said to discuss how people are, what to be studied in humans, and how it should be studied. Studies by Sigmund Freud stated that people would get a cure by making their unconscious thoughts conscious. He also stated that people would also get motivated, which would make them gain great insight into how the human body works.

Later on, psychology changed to analyzing reasons why people behave as they do.. It would research changes in human beings, the psychodynamic, behavioral changes, as well as humanistic and cognitive perspectives. I have discussed the approaches in detail.

Biological Approach

The bio-psychologists normally study how one's nervous system, hormones and how one's genetics may affect one's behavior. They will normally evaluate the connection between one's mental state, their brain and nerves, as well as hormones, which helps them to determine why one thinks as they do; why their mood keeps changing, and why they act the way they do.

What's the meaning of this? According to the biological approach, one is normally equal to their parts. All the thoughts we have on our minds are as a result of how the brain is put together. It is also because of the necessities of the body. The choices that one makes are dependent on the demands of one's body. Through this approach, one is able to get an understanding of the brain and keep it healthy. The mind and the body are also examined in order to find out why some people experience disorders, such as Schizophrenia. A psychologist is able to determine whether it develops through genes, or if the disorder can happen to anyone naturally.

Psychodynamic Approach

This approach was derived from Sigmund Freud, whose belief was that people's impulses are normally determined by sex. He believed that it is through the unconscious involvements that people experience from an early age that cause people to behave the way they do. He stated that when there are societal restrictions on those urges, people are likely to experience conflicts in their behavior. Most psychologists dismissed Sigmund Freud's claims, but there are many times that we experienced this when we are grown-ups, and related them to when we were young kids. This can only mean that Freud's theories are still valid.

Behavioral Approach

This approach states that the environment around us has a great influence on how we behave. It also states that one's behavior is something that can be shaped into the desired behavior. This means that people can be given some training in order for them to be able to act in a particular manner. For people to learn certain behaviors, reinforcements must be used. There are those people who would need to be punished for some kind of behavior to be instilled. They would need to be corrected in a firm way in order for behavior to be instilled in them.

Most people tend to understand the behavioral approach better, since it is normally their day-to-day lives. The people shaping certain behavior do not care much about what people around them might say. All they care about is making sure that those people acquire the behavior they desire. This is the best approach so far as it relates to real-life experiences. How people react to issues and things around them is determined by the behavior they have acquired, and also the behavior that has been instilled in them.

Cognitive Approach

This approach is different from all the above approaches. The cognitive approach states that people will always remember the things that they are already aware of. These are things that people already have some knowledge about. Jean Piaget states that people are able to solve the problems they are experiencing, by remembering things that happened in the past and the experiences they had at that time. Through this approach, people do not get stressed much since they relate the things that they are going through, to whatever happened in the past, and find comfort in the issues.

Humanistic Approach

Humanistic psychologists state that people are normally motivated. They have the potential to achieve everything they would want to achieve in life. They mainly discuss ways of ensuring that people feel good about their achievements, which enables them to be confident and make the most of their time. By utilizing all the time, they have to do the best in various areas, to achieve the best. This enables them to accomplish their set goals, which in return makes them more focused, as they are motivated by the achievements they make.

People are able to get motivation from the people around them. When they are appreciated, they get motivated and even strive to do better in their area. This means that humanistic approaches' main aim is to make sure that people are empowered, and that they achieve their goals in life. It helps in making sure that all the choices you make are helpful in improving your life. This approach does not pressure people to change their lives instantly. It encourages people to work on the areas they are weak in, bit by bit, until they achieve positive results.

Humanitarian psychologists will normally help people take their time to study their behavior, analyze it and come up with reasons why they could be behaving the way they do when faced with certain issues. By finding out the reasons, they are able to look for a remedy, and make sure that they get rid of the behavior.

All these approaches are helpful since they all cover different areas. They, therefore, help in handling the behavior of different people since different people are experiencing different challenges in their behavior.

Chapter 2: How to Analyze People with Psychology

A qualified psychologist should have the ability to analyze people, and be able to come up with a report about their behavior. They should be able to analyze people's behaviors through the knowledge and skills they acquired when undergoing training. With time, they also get experience through the cases they handle in their daily lives. The experience is very useful, as it helps to ensure that one handles the cases that they get, successfully. The experience is also vital in handling different cases since different people have different behaviors.

There are different types of psychologists. They are expected to make sure that they research the areas they handle in order to ensure that they have all the information required to observe various psychological issues. The psychologists should have the desired skills and expertise in order for them to handle all the cases, successfully.

The psychologists are supposed to ensure that they find all the solutions required for people to be able to overcome the challenges they may be facing. They need to handle people as individuals since they all have unique challenges. This will help in ensuring that they analyze their behavior and mental state, without comparing them to others. It is by doing this that they are able to achieve accurate results, which enable them to help them resolve all their behavioral problems.

Researchers state that one can be able to read one's mind, feeling and thoughts. They would, however, be expected to ensure that they have sharp perception skills, which would help them achieve their goal of analysis. Below are some of the ways that psychologists use to analyze people.

Objective And Open-Minded: For a psychologist to be able to read people's minds, they should be able to have an open mind themselves. They should not let their past opinions about people influence their opinion presently. A Psychologist should be able to avoid being biased when analyzing people. This will help them give the correct results for the analysis.

Researchers state that being logical cannot help you to tell the whole story about a person. One has to understand other areas of individuals for them to be able to read other non-verbal signs about an individual. This means that as you analyze, you should be able to listen to the information they give you, and be neutral about it without judging the information. By being neutral, you will be able to get all the information about an individual.

Being open-minded will help people to be able to trust you. There are people who cannot open up to just anybody. They have to trust someone in order for them to give out information. This means that when they learn that a psychologist is biased, they will not trust them with the correct information. The psychologist will, therefore, get the wrong information about an individual.

There are also people who will trust you and open up, because of sharing personal experiences with them. They will express more freely, when they are shown that you can also open up to them, without any fear. This helps a lot since the psychologist will be able to get all the information that you would need.

Appearance: It is important to pay attention to what people are wearing, and even their hairstyle. There are people who will dress up in a certain way when they are sad and also when they are happy. This means that their way of dressing determines their mood. By just having a look at such people, one can be able to tell how they feel.

The appearance of someone when you meet them will tell you a lot. There are people who will dress smart when going for an appointment, while others, will go in any outfit. This says that between the two people, one is cautious while the other does not care at all. A psychologist will be able to tell the type of people they are dealing with, through the way they dress to certain occasions.

Someone's dress code also determines one's personality. People will wear clothing that represents who they are. For example, a Rastafarian will wear clothes that represent them. There are also those who dress according to their religion. This means that a psychologist will be able to learn something from their way of dressing, even before they interact with them. It is important to ensure that when one is addressing people, they try to understand them. By doing this, they will be able to get the right information from them. One should not judge people before they even listen to them.

When one decided to talk to a psychologist, and the psychologist keeps making assumptions through their appearance, they will get bored and may even refuse to cooperate with them. They will feel like there is no need to open up to them anyway.

Posture: How someone sits when you are addressing them tells a lot about their attitude. When talking to someone who holds their head high, it will tell you that they are confident. The way they answer questions will also tell you whether they are ready to give information about them or not. There are those that will just stare at you when you talk to them, while there are those who will answer you immediately.

There are also people who will walk as they cower, and without conviction. These kinds of people may be experiencing low self-esteem, who do not believe in themselves. They are people who feel shy and may not be able to speak to people outright. They may have a lot of fear about a lot of things, and so they may fear to disclose them to people. This makes it hard for a psychologist to derive information from them.

These kinds of people have to trust you enough in order for them to give you any information about them. It is therefore important for a psychologist to understand these kinds of people and take their time when talking to them, in order for them to get the right information, which will be of great help in the analysis. Psychologists should make sure that all their clients are able to communicate with them without experiencing any challenges. They can even start the conversation by asking simple questions about the clients, and questions about the things that they are familiar with.

By doing that, they will help people to feel free to discuss issues with them, without fear. They will also be able to sit well and pay attention to them, which will help you as a psychologist to achieve the set goals.

Watching Their Physical Movements: There are people who express their feelings about themselves through the movements that they make. One example is that we will lean on someone that we like, and will lean away from the people that we do not like. There are also people who will cross their hands to show that they are angry and arrogant; also those who will cross their hands as a way to show that they are self-protecting themselves.

People who leave their hands free are selfless. They are not complicated and are easy to talk to and interact with. One will also be able to easily approach them, and you will be able to talk to them easily. You will observe that others bite their lips or their cuticles. This is a sign of soothing oneself. It means that they face their challenges through comforting themselves. These kinds of people are interactive, but they can also keep things to themselves. A psychologist should make sure that they come up with ways of ensuring that they handle them with care, in order for them to be able to give out the required information.

Interpret Facial Expressions: Facial expressions are the easiest to read when having a discussion with someone. People react to different situations through their facial expressions. When you ask someone a question, the first facial expression is how he or she feels about the question. If they smile, then they have taken the question positively, if they hold back or frown then they took the question negatively.

Since people are different, there are those who will frown at the mention of certain things while there are those who will smile at that exact thing. Frowning may be a sign that one is sad or maybe overthinking various situations. A frown may also be a sign of discomfort about certain issues. A psychologist should be able to read these expressions, and know how to handle them in order for them to be able to understand them, and get some information about them.

Someone will smile at situations that make the person happy. A psychologist will, therefore, be able to read their expressions, and be able to tell whether it is the right time to question them or not. The best time to question and analyze them is when they are happy. This is because they will be honest about their thoughts and feelings.

There are three types of smiles. One of them being a reward smile. This is a type of smile that communicates that one will have positive feedback. Positive feedback is very important when a psychologist is analyzing people. When one shows a reward smile, it shows that they are likely to give honest feedback, which is helpful when a psychologist is doing some analysis. It will be helpful since the psychologist will be able to get all the information, they may require a certain individual.

There is also the affiliate smile. This kind of smile is given as a sign of friendship or liking. Someone will give this smile to show that they like you, and that they would want to be friends with you. When someone shows the affiliate smile, the psychologist should take advantage of it and make friends with these people. This will help him to be able to make friends with them and in return be able to analyze them without experiencing any challenges.

Encouraging Small Talk: Small talks are very important when a psychologist is analyzing people. The psychologist can initiate small talks about the weather, how the client's day was, how they think their day will end and any other kinds of questions that would make the conversation to keep moving. The small talks enable them to be able to know people more, which in return helps you to be able to understand them. The small talks are useful in enabling you as a psychologist to observe one's behavior.

These small talks help you to learn how people behave in their normal situations. You will be able to discover the things that annoy them and those that make them happy. This is of great help since one will be able to observe the difference when they change their behavior. The psychologists normally use the small talks for benchmarking. They are therefore able to spot any unusual behavior easily.

Scanning Overall Behavior:

People behave differently all the time. They will show one behavior today and show a different one the next day. This is because they may be in different environments each day. The psychologists will, therefore, be able to study people's behavior patterns. This will give them an insight into how people behave each time they experience changes in their lives. By doing this, they will be able to have a better understanding of what annoys them, and what makes them happy. The analysis is made easy since a psychologist has studied their behavior patterns, and understood them even better.

Asking Questions That Give Straight Answers: A psychologist should ensure that they ask straight questions in order for them to get straight answers. The questions they ask should help in analyzing people. Straight questions do not give people room to think about other issues apart from the questions asked. They should, therefore, ensure that once they ask questions, they do not interrupt them when they are answering you. This will help a lot in ensuring that you get all the information being given. The information is useful in analyzing their behavior, since you will be able to learn how they behave through the questions.

Interrupting people when they are answering you will also make them forget some points. They will give answers to points that they remember, which means that there is some information that you will miss out on.

Take Note Of The Tone Used: As the psychologist is talking to people, they should be able to notice the tone they used when they are discussing various issues. They should make sure that they notice where different tones are used when talking about the issues affecting them.

There are people who rely on how you ask questions, in order for them to know how they will answer you. They observe your attitude, which dictates how they will answer your questions. They're also people who need to be praised for them to feel good about themselves, and in return, they will give all the information that you require. It is therefore important for a psychologist to learn different people, and how they react to different things. They need to also learn the things that would make them talk in order for them to use them in their analysis.

Avoid Assumptions: Most of the time, assumptions make people experience misunderstandings with the psychologist. When a psychologist assumes various things about someone, they will cause the person to hold back, and when they do, they are not honest about the information they give. People cannot cooperate with someone who keeps assuming things about them. They will find them annoying. Some may just choose to listen to them without answering their questions.

Psychologists also use the perspectives of psychology to analyze people. There are five approaches that enable the psychologist to be able to analyze people successfully. They have been discussed below and how they help in analyzing people.

Biological Approach

A biological approach is used when a psychologist is looking at some of the psychological issues that may be affecting someone. By finding out the psychological issues affecting people, one is able to tell the reasons why they behave the way they behave. Psychologists should ensure that they take their time when studying human behavior, in order for them to get the best results.

Researchers have stated that through the study of physiology and also biological issues, one is able to differentiate the behaviors that are a result of genetics from those that have been acquired as a result of the environment that people are living in. Charles Darwin was the first researcher to discuss evolution, and stating that genetics play a great role in one's behavior. There are people who inherit some of the behaviors they have from their parents and other relatives. Acquired behaviors are hard to change. This is because one is born with it, unlike the behaviors that people acquire from the environment they are living in.

Charles Darwin stated that most of the behaviors that are said to help people continue surviving, are the ones that are mostly passed on from one generation to another. Those that are dangerous are mostly not passed down to other people. Through the biological approach, a psychologist is able to study and understand the problems that people encounter in their daily lives. They are able to analyze the problems, their causes, which enable them to understand the reasons why people have a certain behavior.

There are people who might show some aggression from when they were children, while there are those who develop the problem as they grow up. It may be difficult to eliminate that issue when they have grown up with it, but it is very easy to change one's behavior once it is noted early enough. Through the behavioral approach, it is easy to shape one's behavior through reinforcement, and also through punishments. Those with good behavior may reinforce it by making sure that they keep doing well while those whose behavior is negative might need to be punished for them to improve their behavior. Once the psychologists discover the cause for the behaviors, they will be able to help individuals get rid of it.

The bio-psychologists analyze so many things, even though their interest, in how the biological forces help in shaping people's behavior. They analyze the following things.

• Analyzing the way in which trauma may be influencing one's behavior.

• Analyzing how the degenerative parts of brain illnesses affect people's actions.

• Finding out how genetics influence people's behaviors.

• Discovering how one's genetics and brain damage cause them to experience mental disorders.

There are very many advantages of using the biological approach to analyze behavior. One of them is that it is normally very scientific. Most of the things that are scientific give results that are reliable and dependable. The results are also said to be practical, which makes the bio-psychologists get firsthand information about every required detail.

It is also through biological research that people have been able to discover a treatment for different kinds of diseases, which are psychological. This has helped people to feel better, since the treatments ease their pain and ensure that they live their lives without stressing the people around them.

Cognitive Approach

Psychologists normally use a cognitive approach since it is used in the study of people's minds, which is also said to be a processor of information. The psychologists study everything that goes through people's minds. They study people's perception of issues facing them, the things they give full attention to, their language and memory, their thinking and also how much their mind is conscious.

Through a cognitive approach, psychologists are able to study people's minds, and are able to find out the things that may be affecting them. This is because they could be the reason for them to behave and act the way they do. Many people may have underlying issues, but may not talk about them. When they fail to share them, they may find themselves developing mental issues that could have been avoided.

It is the work of psychologists to analyze people's mental state, which will help them to ensure that they discover some of the challenges they may be going through early enough. Psychologists state that one's brain works like a computer. The process is complicated, but yet very efficient when it comes to the processing of the information in the brain.

Psychologists are said to have adopted information, processing ideas for them to learn how the human brain works. When information is being processed, there are assumptions that are developed by psychologists. They include:

•   The information that is available in one's immediate environment is normally processed through a sequence of some processing systems. These processes include people's attention, their perception towards things and short-term memory.

•   The processing systems are said to distort any given information in a very systematic manner.

•   It is also clear that information processing in human beings is normally similar to the processes of a computer.

The cognitive approach is said to produce results that are very efficient. This is because psychologists are able to discover reasons why people behave as they do. They are also able to find treatment for people with mental problems, and ensure that they get the right medication. This causes individuals to live a normal life, which is free from challenges.

Behavioral Approach

This type of approach is said to deal with the behavior itself. The psychologists specialize in finding out reasons as to why individuals behave in a particular manner. They make sure that they take their time to observe people's behavior. They may interrogate the people they are analyzing in order for them to understand them, and their reasons for behaving the way they do. There are very many people who may be struggling with mental issues and do not understand where they stem from. A psychologist strives to understand people and reasons why they have problems with their brains.

Through the analysis of behavior, one is able to discover people's weaknesses and strengths. They will be able to help people to deal with their weaknesses, which in return, cause them to regain their esteem and confidence. Through that, they will be able to interact with people around them without any challenges. They are also able to help other people who may deal with the same issues they were dealing with.

The psychologists may also help people to realize their abilities. They help them discover them and work towards making themselves better. The people with disabilities benefit from this most, since they are enabled to become more active, such that most of them are able to depend on themselves. They will not have to depend on the people around them, in order to perform various activities.

The psychologists analyze behavior in different ways. They include:

- Through experimenting with people's behavior.

- Through analyzing practical behavior.

- Through analyzing theoretical behavior.

For the researchers to be able to analyze behavior successfully, they have to analyze some facts about certain behavior and try to understand it. After analyzing it, they still have to analyze it practically, in order for them to come up with the correct results. They have to ensure that after carrying out the research, they come up with ways of changing the behavior and make sure that the behavior is changed.

It is clear that through behaviorism, children who have had challenges with autism and delays in their development have been able to get help through this approach. They have been enabled to acquire helpful skills, which they use in their daily lives. This has helped them to be able to stop being dependent on people for them to carry out their usual activities.

Psychodynamic Approach

This approach describes ways in which one functions, even as they interact with forces that are within them. It mostly analyzes the unconscious parts of the brain. The unconscious parts of the brain are the mental progressions that are normally not accessible. The conscious parts of the brain are those that influence people to become judgmental, have feelings towards things, and also which make people show certain behavior.

Though the Psychodynamic Approach, psychologists are able to understand that some of the behaviors that people have were acquired when they were children. This helps them understand its origin, and look for ways to get rid of it. This helps when it comes to shaping people's personalities. This is because they begin by helping them let go of the challenges that they have experienced in the past, which in return enables them to slowly enable them to make their behavior better.

The psychologists believe that all our behaviors have a cause. They also believe that most of the behaviors we have in our adulthood are as a result of our childhood experiences. They are therefore able to handle people with behavioral problems successfully by eliminating their past behaviors and dealing with the current problems that they may be experiencing.

It is therefore important for psychologists to ensure that they understand people's past before they judge their behavior. This will help in ensuring that they deal with all the problems at once, and ensure that they do not keep recurring.

Chapter 3: Psychology's Applied Fields

Recent Developments In Psychology

If there is an ever-evolving field it is psychology, there are several types of research that have been conducted over the years. The research conducted offers explanations, and establishes the recent developments of psychology. Below are some of the recent developments in the field of psychology.

Mentality–Body Merge

There is always a connection between emotional health and physical health. According to new research conducted, they found the new form of therapy. The new energy psychology was created to combine mind-body therapy and the self-help method. This method was developed by dividing the developments into different areas, such as medicine and psychology, as well as chiropractic and the kinesiology. Though you will find that most of the psychologist will try and pay attention to health issues by finding ways to deal with both emotional and physical health.

Evaluating Mental Health

Before they start administering any medication, they should try finding out what could be the problem. Some have come with a standardized measuring scale to measure anxiety and anger. If the same can be done to the mental health sector, then we will be in the position to find out the degree of mental sickness and emotions. The standardized scale can be of great help. If this could be used the impact will be felt by the patients.

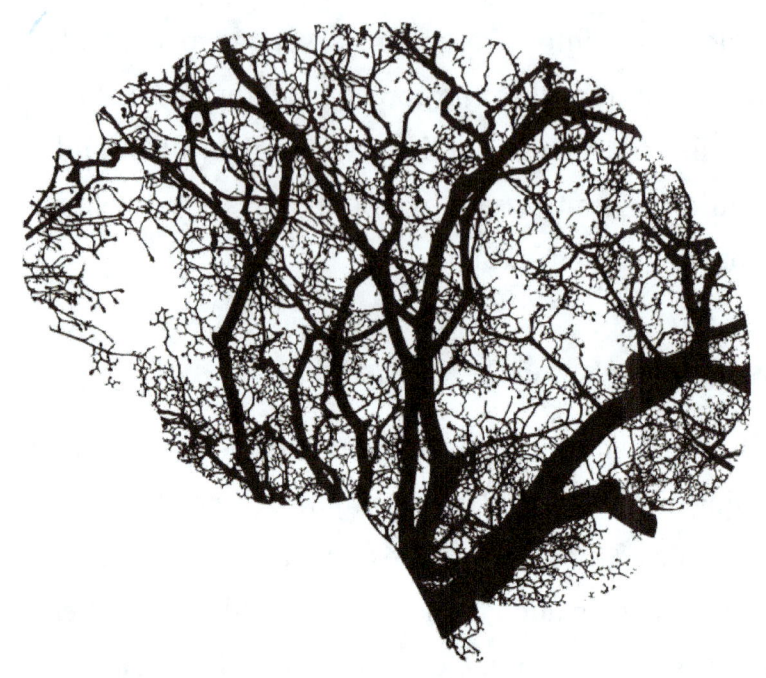

Behavioral Financial Side

This field of psychology deals with people if they want to buy something; they buy what they already identified in the field. This psychology tends to look into why we prefer some things, over others. Could it be the driving force of the pressure out there? Could it be we buy because they appeal in the eyes of one? That could be the major reason why people don't make decisions on what they want, but buy them because they look appealing.

Knowing a Problem

What could be the cause of mental illness? This is the area that has been newly focused by the researchers. They are trying to identify if it could be an environmental cause, or situations that could cause future problems. For instance, a parent who had a mental illness, such as bipolar condition; the child may likely develop the same condition or another psychiatric condition.

Evolving Field

Research is being conducted all over the world by thousands of psychologists. We have the constant publication of psychology articles, which has brought changes to the face of psychology.

Psychotherapy And Counseling

Psychotherapy and counseling are often considered therapies that do the work of guiding one when depressed, or while going through hard times. But there are some important differences between the two. When you have been recommended that you visit a counselor, you might be undergoing specific issues, such drug addiction or grieving, and the process will take barely weeks to months. While when one is told to visit psychotherapist, he will try and explore past issues, which may be contributing to the present problem. This process will take place continuously over a period of years. In other cases, you will find that the two processes will overlap, and will help the patient to get well faster.

The two are used to describe professionals who used the same approach of talk-based therapy, to try helping someone recover from mental health and mental illness. When undergoing a hard situation, it is good to talk to someone. People may find that talking to a friend or a family member will help them feel better. A professional counselor and therapist will offer more, because of the skills they acquired in training. They are more experienced because they have handled more issues. They also create emotional distance, since they don't know so much about you, they only know that you are their client. They will use different theories to listen to the client, giving support and handling different problems.

There are many psychotherapists with good experience, who know which approach to use when dealing with certain issues. The therapy and counseling are the same no matter what approach you prefer to use, the expectation incur is having an understanding of the problem, though the therapist; as well as the trust, you have now built between each other. This will bring a 100% improvement in the patient.

It is good to understand the differences that exist between the two when having a problem, you know who to visit when having such a case. You will have chosen an effective method to deal with your situation. The two can provide counseling and psychotherapy, but a psychotherapist is more equipped with more skills than a counselor. Those who conduct psychotherapy are trained professionals either on psychotherapists or psychologists. The psychotherapist is qualified to provide counseling. For the counselor, he is trained or may not be trained but he is in a position to give counseling. A counselor may not be in a position to provide the psychotherapeutic functions to a patient, because in his area of training he did not train as a psychotherapist.

Counseling

A counselor means an advisor; they offer short term treatment. The counseling process involves two people, the counselor and the one taking the advice, or the patient. The two people work together to solve a problem. Advice is given based on the situation faced by the patient. In a case where we have a patient suffering from mental health, he was recommended that he visit a counselor. The counselor will try and offer guidance and support, as the patient tries to figure out ways to manage and accept the changes that he may be going through in life. There are many types of counselors such as drug addictions, grief counselors, family and marriage.

Psychotherapy

This is a long-term treatment offered to patients; the therapist tries to gain the impending, chronic disease whether it be a physical or emotional problem. The treatment focuses on the patient's thinking process, and how the process was influenced by past events and may end up causing the current problem. The therapist identifies the root cause of the problem, and the core factors that have contributed to the present. We have several types of psychotherapy, which include cognitive behavioral therapy, dialectic therapy and many more.

Similarities

We have many similarities between psychotherapy and counseling. They include the development of the healing process, which is safe because of the relationship between the patient and the therapist. They are both health care providers who assess the condition of the patient and determine the state of the mind. The two methods are very effective for both children and adults. The therapist is in a position of understanding the patients' feelings and behaviors, and they will always have the aim of improving the lives of the patient. Both the counseling and the psychotherapy require that the therapist should have highly developed skill. They should have undergone training for a couple of years before they offer their services to the patients. They should also be under supervision from the practitioners.

Differences

Are there major differences between counseling and psychotherapy? The reason could be because they are both used interchangeably there is an overlap in some instances.

The counseling process is a secondary process that focuses on the current. situation, and they deal with the specific situation and behaviors. Their therapy takes a short period of weeks to not more than six months. They focus on the actions of the patients and behaviors. It involves a lot of talking, dialogue between two people. The therapist gives guidance, they also give support and education to help the patients to identify their problem, and also finding a solution to the problems they are going through.

The psychotherapy process is a primary process, which focuses on the chronic and recurrent situation. They also try to get the overall pattern of the chronic situation, and how it has gotten itself the big picture. The therapy will take a very long time, and the process is continuous over the years. They focus on the feelings and the experience of the patient to establish the problem. There is carried out testing to establish the personality and intelligence and other types of therapists may be included. They focus more on the internal thinking and feelings, which has led to personal growth.

Psychotherapist or Counselor

How will you choose between the psychotherapist and a counselor? They only way you can choose between the counselor and the psychotherapist is by first knowing the differences that exist between the two. Know what each provides and the approaches that they use. At some point, the choice will depend on whom you prefer to see, and the accessibility of the two. The most important part is who do you trust with your secrets, then you can get to that person, and try to share your problems.

When should one see a counselor? One may be in a position to see a counselor if the situation he/she wishes to address is a short-term problem. The patient may also wish to know how to cope with such conditions, and better their future and life, as well. When one has had a divorce, they can seek advice from a counselor on how to cope in such a scenario. Someone who is addicted and is trying to live without the drugs can also seek help from the counselor. What they are looking for is a coach who is going to guide, support and educates you on how to survive, and help you recognize the problem and try giving you solutions to your problem.

When should one see the psychotherapist? One may be in a better position to see a psychotherapist when the situation he is going through has impacted negatively on the relationship and life as well. When you are battling with trauma, and a situation from the past is playing a role in the current situation. The issues the person is undergoing keeps recurring, and they are now chronic. When one had seen a counselor, with no improvement at all, that would be the point to see a psychotherapist.

Should we treat depression through the use of counseling or psychotherapy? Yes, both are used in the treatment of depression. One's choice will depend on the nature of depression, either chronic or has been a short time since the problem began. From the several types of research that have been conducted, it is found that counseling can be effective to treat moderate depression. Those with chronic, severe depression will have to see a psychotherapist.

People have varied reasons why they wish to choose between counselors, instead of a psychotherapist or vice versa. The reason behind it can be trust, getting that particular person you can trust to help you with the situation you are facing. That could be the reason most people move from one to the other, until they get to the right therapist.

How Does Psychotherapy Work?

Psychotherapy is used to find the main cause of frustrations. It is assumed that what causes depression in the present time is what might have happened in the past. In some other instances, it may be hard to know if whatever you are going through could be related to what happened in the past. For some of the individuals, they may not be in a position to know that trauma is caused by past events which will have negative impacts and the current decisions and behavior. The psychotherapist will come in with his skills and try to use many therapies. The process relies on the patient and the therapist, they need to have an understanding of which therapies to apply to the patient. They use behavioral therapy, modification of the behavior of the patient, mindful-based and not forgetting the insight-oriented therapy. The therapist will pick a method after making the diagnosis of the patient and know what could be the needs of the patient. That is the reason the patient and the therapist should have a good rapport.

How Does Counseling Work?

The effectiveness of counseling depends on the relationship between the counselor and the patient. You will only achieve in counseling if you use the talk therapy to help the client work through the issues that harm their life. The counselors have to listen, give feedback, and try to provide advice. The counselor does not give the client answers but facilitates the process of finding answers. The counselors only discus the current behaviors and will help you to understand why those behaviors are unwanted. They will ask questions to try and understand some of the situations in your life. When asking this question, he will be busy trying to read your thinking process. When the counselor has known much about you then the counseling process becomes easy. When planning to visit a counselor bare in your mind that you must be prepared to be honest about your personal life. You should also include all the recent changes that you may have experienced. What could be more important is expressing what you may be feeling inside you?

Why Do People Need Psychotherapy?

People get to see the psychotherapist because they can be having a problem with their mental health or have a problem with their emotions. The psychotherapist will help such people to eliminate and being in a position to control such symptoms so that he can function again as the whole person. Psychotherapy is a wide range of treatments that can be ministered to those with mental health problems, those with emotional challenges and those with a psychiatric disorder. People have a wide range of problems; they range from fear of maybe taking a flight to big ones such as depressions. Some of the reasons you may seek help from the psychotherapy are:

When Having Chronic Emotional Agony

Going through emotional agony is normal since it is part of our life. At times, this agony tends to be more severe and can take long before a solution can be found it can even result in impairing your life. Therapy can help you if you feel distressed and the distress can persist and sometimes you will not have the peace of mind that you require, you will always be troubled.

Relationship Problems

When having difficulty in a relationship it contributes to emotional distress. The difficult relationship can be from a spouse, child, co-worker, and other people we live around. Therapy may be of help since you will be able to understand the reasons why you are depressed which will enable you to look for treatment early enough. Some of the relationships are connected to a deficiency in a certain skill. Such issues may include being shy, lack of confidence, lack of communication skills and poor way of controlling your anger. The therapy sections will enable you to improve on these skills and acquire better skills to deal with life. The treatment will focus on affecting them with the correct skill to be able to make them feel better.

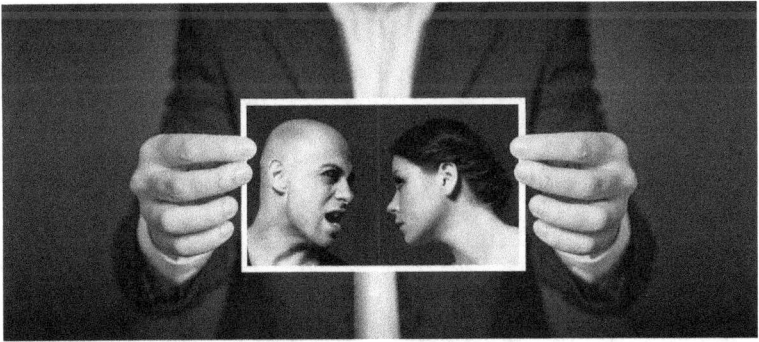

Loss

Loss can happen to anyone, be it death snatching away someone who was so close to you or having a separation from someone you adored. Enduring such breaks can be a bit hard for one. It may even affect the way of his life. It will result in great emotional pain. Therapy will be in a position to help you cope with the loss.

Sexual Problems

Such problems may be dissatisfaction or dysfunction. These are common among married couples and may feel embarrassed to talk about such issues. The therapist will help you to get back to the journey of the two obtaining the most enjoyment out of the sexual functioning.

Trauma or Abuse

When one has been a victim of being abused physically or sexually or any other way of violence can happen to anyone, we are all affected. You may have had an accident in a vehicle that has left scars in your body or left you unable to do some of the work yourself. The psychotherapy will create room for you to be able to discuss while they offer the support and care that you may require to be able to live a better life again. They will focus on helping you heal all the wounds left by the accident. They will see to it that you will be able to move forward with your life.

Personal Growth

It is not that you have a medical condition that you should see the psychotherapist but you can see the therapist when you want to get some advice or any teachings on how you can be able to take control of your issues and all the things that happen in your life. It can help you to deal with the complications that have delayed you from the attainment of your goals and above all, being able to become the person you have always wanted to become.

Clinical Disorder

A person with a mental disorder can also see the psychotherapist and other forms of conditions such as major depression and bipolar disorder. They will not only get the therapy sections but also, they will undergo some medication. If the two won't be combined then the treatment won't bare the positive results.

The psychotherapy is a safe process where no one is supposed to judge your story, you will have to share everything with the professional who is trained to help you. The major benefits of seeing a psychotherapist are that you will learn more about your mental health and emotions. The work of the therapist will be to listen to you and try to connect your experiences. After that, they may opt to offer guidance and make recommendations where necessary. They will not tell you what you are supposed to do but they only guide you. It is now your own choice to make your actions. If you are not realistic about the goals you have set then you can visit the psychotherapy where he will offer help to you to clarify the goals and set realistic goals that will make you achieve your goals.

If you are in a relationship or not the therapy can make you have a fulfilling relationship. The therapy will try and address issues of difficulty I relating to others, insecurity in a relationship and issues to do with trust. If you visit the psychotherapy you will tend to have a better life and health. There is a link between the mind and the wellness of the body. The untreated mental condition can cause effects on the physical body. Those who are well emotionally can handle any kind of health issues that may come up. Through therapy, people will be able to experience improvement in their lives. Whenever you feel like there are some things that may be holding you back from reaching your goals, you can always look for help from therapists and they will be of great help to you. There are those times when you may not really be sure about the things that may be holding you back. It would be advisable to look for help from people around you or from a therapist.

You don't just wake up one day and you decide you are visiting psychotherapy, but it takes some considerations. May be your condition keeps showing different signs. You may want to give it more time and see it is improving or not. You need to see a therapist if you have an issue that causes distress and has interfered with your life. Especially when you have soothing that bothers for an hour while you try finding a solution. If the problem will cause embarrassment or make you avoid people close to you, it will be clear that the issues you may be experiencing may have weighed you down. It also means that your life has been affected negatively. If you have all those experiences then you need to see the therapist. The therapy process will help you to reduce the impact.

This treatment aims to make the patients know their feeling and what makes them feel positive, anxious, or depressed. This makes them have the necessary knowledge on how to cope with whatever conditions they may be having. The process takes a minimum of a year at that point the patient who wants positive results at the end of the process will be more willing to learn from the psychotherapist. The type of help provided by the therapist cut across all types of psychotherapy ranging from depression to family disputes. People benefit from the process and with a combination of medication.

Who will benefit from the psychotherapy process? Those who have been overwhelmed by the feeling of sadness become helpless when it comes to life. Those who have daily problems and are unable to cope with such problems are considered fit for the process. The people when finding it hard to concentrate at work or at studies most of the time is fit for the process of psychotherapy. Those who drink too much, taking drugs to the extent of putting their lives in danger and those of their friends are also considered fit for the process. Those with problems which seem that the problems never seem to get better even though they have received help from friends and supportive family members.

How effective is the method? This is the process of making one understand himself or herself. The patient has the benefit of having someone he can talk to. It is a way of trying to look for a solution to a difficult situation. Those who have understood themselves will have an improved relationship. For this process to work the patient must participate actively either during sessions or after the session and practicing new skills. People may also need to see a psychotherapist because they have a problem in which it is impacting their lives on the negative side. A person may have been under trauma that experience he had has been traumatizing him in the present life. a person may be having a mental health condition. That particular person has to see the psychotherapist. A person, who has seen a counselor yet her issues are not improving at all, got to see a psychotherapist so that she can get help from him.

Psychotherapy has been proven to have worked from the research which has conducted. The research shows that the individuals who had symptoms have shown signs of relief and are doing better in their lives.

There are different types of psychotherapy. The therapist will try and use the approach after he has made the diagnosis of the condition you will be suffering from. Each approach used is like a road map to find out what the client may be suffering from and after that provide a solution to the condition. The kind of medication you will receive will depend on a variety of factors. They will narrow down to the analysis of the research, theoretical orientations and lastly what will work best for the problem.

The theoretical orientation is affected by what happens in the office of the therapist. The approach used will depend on the conditions of the client. The cognitive and behavioral is a practical approach to treating. The therapist will ask you to tackle a certain task that will help you to cope with the condition you are suffering from. The approach involves homework. The therapist may require you to find better ways you can deal with the condition you may be suffering from. He may want you to use the acquired skill between the sessions so that he may see how you are coping with the new skill. He may also give you the reading assignments to help you to learn about a particular topic.

The psychoanalytic and humanistic approach focuses more on talking than the practical part. You will find that the psychotherapist spending all sessions discussing the earlier experience that will help the therapist to establish the root cause of your problems. The therapist will combine different styles of skills from psychotherapy and try to give treatment by blending several possible approaches to provide medication. The therapist will not concentrate on one approach. What is important to know if the therapist has more knowledge in the area you are supposed to be helped?

Chapter 4: Psychology of Personality

We often talk of personality or at least hear other people talk about it. Many of us cannot describe it scientifically, because we do not understand fully what the psychological study of personality is all about. Regardless of having a rough idea of what personality is, we still find the question, "what is personality?" lingering in our minds. Understanding our own personality helps us to gain more insight into our emotional wellbeing and improve our interpersonal relationships.

Every one of us has a unique personality. It is our personality that makes us who we are and influences our relationships with others, our overall wellbeing, and the way we look at life in general.

Personality psychology is a branch of psychology that seeks to understand personality, in terms of how individuals are different or similar due to psychological forces. How personality develops, and its influence in the way we behave and think is what psychologists strive to understand in personality psychology. Studies in this large and popular branch of psychology touch on different psychological disorders that interfere with an individual's day to day life, their assessment, diagnosis, and treatment. In this chapter, we are going to look at various types of psychological disorders, but before we delve in, lets us look at what exactly is personality.

What Is Personality?

Personality entails character patterns, behavior, feelings, and thoughts that contribute to an individual's uniqueness. An individual's personality arises from within and relatively remains constant throughout their entire life. All the social attitudes, thoughts, and behavior patterns that affect ones' believe of self, and the way they view others and the surrounding world encompass one's personality. It is your personality that makes you who you are, and factors such as your life experiences, your genetics, environment, and upbringing contribute to the kind of person you are. In other words, these factors determine your personality. Your personality determines how you respond or react to different situations and the things you value and prefer.

Psychology of personality is a vast subject and touches on various aspects that make us who we are. Psychologists use different ways to think and understand personality. They may focus on individual traits, or look at various developmental stages over time, as personality emerges and change sometimes. In this field, psychologists' concern is not just to understand the healthy human character, but also to recognize potential psychological disorders and other disturbances that lead to difficulties and distress in crucial areas of life such as school, relationships, and work. With such understanding, they can help people develop the necessary skillset, to manage, adapt, and cope with the symptoms of various psychological disturbances. Without a doubt, then, the psychology of personality is a very import field.

Personality Disorders

A personality disorder is a long-term pattern of behavior, way of thinking, and inner feelings or experience that deviate significantly from what is expected. These are some of the disorders associated with personality.

- **Antisocial Personality Disorder:** a person with this disorder disregards and violates the rights of others. He may deceive or lie to others repeatedly, act impulsively, and go against established social norms.

- **Dependent Personality Disorder:** characterized by cling behavior, submissiveness, and wanting to be taken care of. Such people feel helpless and uncomfortable alone since they feel unable to take care of themselves. They are weak and awkward alone.

- **Avoidant Personality Disorder:** it is characterized by extreme sensitivity to criticism, excessive shyness, and constant feelings of inadequacy. People with avoidant personality disorder tend to avoid getting involved with others unless they are sure to be liked. They are preoccupied with the fear of rejection or criticism. They are not socially inept, and they see themselves as not being good enough.

- **Histrionic Personality Disorder:** characterized by wanting to seek attention and excess emotions. A person with this disorder wants all the attention to be centered on them and get a feeling of discomfort when they are not. They experience exaggerated emotions that shift rapidly and may use physical appearance to draw attention.

- **Borderline Personality Disorder:** a pattern of being impulsive, intense emotions, poor self-image, and instability in relationships. A person with borderline disorder has feelings of emptiness, intense display anger, suicidal attempts, and will go to great lengths to avoid being abandoned.

- **Narcissism:** characterized by lacking empathy for others and unquenchable thirst admiration. Narcissists have a sense of entitlement, take advantage of others, and have an inflated sense of self-worth.

- **Schizotypal:** characterized by acentric behavior,

distorted thinking, and being very uncomfortable in close relationships. A person may experience social anxiety, peculiar beliefs, and strange speech or behavior.

- **Obsessive-Compulsive Personality Disorder:** a character of control, perfectionism, and issuing orders. People with an obsessive-compulsive personality disorder may be inflexible in values and morality and may work excessively with no time for friends or leisure. They are focused on schedules and strict with details.

- **Schizoid Personality Disorder:** expressing little emotion and being detached from social relationships. A person with a schizoid personality disorder doesn't care about criticism or praise from others, chooses to be alone and doesn't seek close relationships

- **Paranoid Personality Disorder:** suspicious of being seen as spiteful or mean by others. People with a paranoid personality disorder do not confide to others or become close to them because they assume, they maybe are deceived or harmed.

Dissociative Disorders

These are mental disorders involving problems with memory, perception behavior, sense of self, and identity. They are characterized by experiencing a lack of continuity, and disconnection between memories, thoughts, actions, surroundings, and behavior. A person with a dissociative disorder will escape reality in an unhealthy and involuntary way. Dissociative symptoms have the potential to interfere with every area of mental functioning and cause troubles in the day to day life. These disorders include:

- **Dissociative Amnesia:** this entails a loss of memory as the familiar sign, which cannot be linked to any medical problem, and whose severity is more than normal forgetfulness. It becomes difficult to remember information about yourself, people close to your life or events, more so from a traumatic time. It may involve specific circumstances, at a particular time, as in the case of intense combat. In rare cases, it can lead to total memory loss on oneself. At times you get confused and get outside oneself. Such episodes happen suddenly and may take a short duration or for an extended period. A continuation of amnesia can take a few minutes or some hours, and in rare cases, it can last for several months and years.

- **Dissociative Identity Disorder:** in this type of

disorder, a person switches to alternative identities. It is also called multiple personality disorder. You feel possessed by other characters. It can happen in such a way that you feel two or more people present in your head, living there and talking to you. Each one of them has a different character and history, a unique name, a distinct voice, and a mixed gender.

- **Depersonalization- Derealization Disorder:** it may involve a continuous or intermitted sense of being detached or getting outside of yourself. It appears as if you are watching your thoughts, feelings, actions, and self from a distance. In the case of depersonalization, you feel as if you a watching movie from a distance. In the case of derealization, you feel detached from people, and things around you, and everything appears to be dreamlike or foggy. Time slows down or gets sped up, and the world doesn't seem to be real. Symptoms are usually distressing and may last for short moments or come and go over a long time.

Symptoms

- Losing memory and forgetting personal information, people close to you or certain events and periods

- A feeling of being detached from your emotions and yourself

- Perceiving the surrounding environment in a distorted and unreal manner

- Enormous problems, work, and relationship-related stress

- Being unable to cope with professional or emotional stress

- Depression, anxiety, suicidal thoughts and behavior, and other mental health problems.

- Two or more distinct identities existing in your head, accompanied by changes in memory, thinking, and behavior

Mood Disorders

Life, being a roller coaster of emotions, comes with changes in moods. One day you feel at the top of the world, because your spouse has showered you with love and gifts, or because you got a promotion at work. Another day you are struggling with financial difficulties, relationships troubles and stress from work, and you feel down in the dumps. These are normal mood swings because they come and go. When your mood gets to the point where it begins to interfere with your daily activities, relationships, and work, then it is no longer healthy, it is a mood disorder.

Mood disorders involve distorted mood or emotional state that is not consistent with your prevailing circumstances and may disrupt your normal functioning and interfere with life activities. A person with mood disorders may become empty, irritable, or extremely sad, or experience periods of depression intermitted by excessive happiness. One's moods can also be affected by anxiety disorders and depression, which can enhance one's risk chances of committing suicide.

There are several mood disorders:

- **Premenstrual Dysphoric Disorder:** this is the irritability and mood changes that happen at a time just before the start of the menstrual cycle in women and disappear when the menses commence.

- **Medical Illness Depression:** a depressed mood that is persistent and comes with a loss of displeasure in most activities. It can be caused by the physical effects of a medical condition.

- **Persistent Depression Disorder:** this is a type of chronic depression that lingers for long. This condition is also called dysthymia

- **Mood Dysregulation:** it is a chronic disorder, where a child experiences severe and persistent irritability. It involves outbursts of temper which occur persistently and are inconsistent with the developmental age of the child.

- **Cyclothymic Disorder:** This disorder occurs when one experiences emotional ups and downs at a lesser degree than bipolar disorder

- **Depression Sparked By Medication Or Substance Use:** these are depression symptoms developing immediately after exposure to medication or after substance use or withdrawal.

- **Major Depressive Disorder:** this is where one

experiences long and continuous durations of unusual sadness

- **Seasonal Affective Disorder (SAD):** it is a depression type that is linked with fewer hours of daylight, especially in the southern and northern latitudes.

- **Bipolar Disorder**: it involves mania and depression occurring alternatingly. It is also known as a bipolar affective disorder or manic depression.

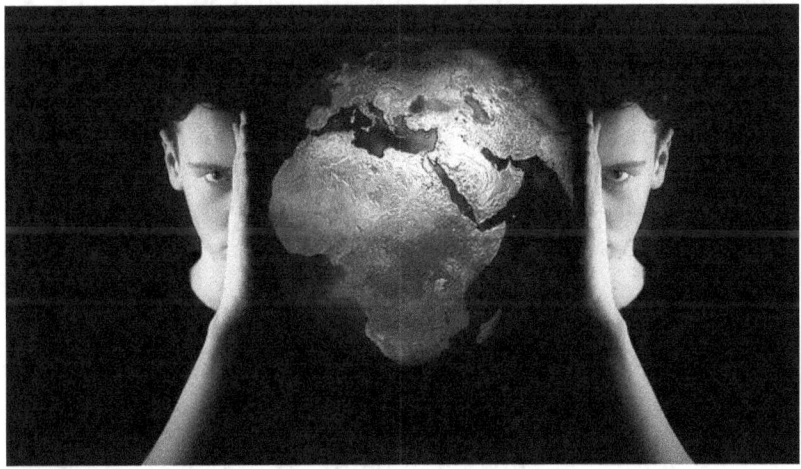

Somatoform Disorders

These entail a set of psychological conditions where and the individual suffers bodily symptoms that cannot be explained or accounted for by a neurological or medical diagnosis. They involve bodily pains and physical sensations which are linked to mental illness. Symptoms vary in severity and range from mild and less frequent, to severe and chronic, usually out of a person's conscious control. They cause a lot of distress and trigger anxious feelings and stress, which impairs everyday functioning. They can make a person take more time contemplating or acting in response to them.

There are different types of somatoform disorders. They include:

- **Somatization Disorder:** a person keeps on complaining about physical symptoms, without any visible physical condition to cause such symptoms. For you to be diagnosed with somatization disorder, it requires experiencing physical symptoms that cannot be explained before the age of thirty, that continue for several years involving pain, neurological problems, sexual issues, and stomach complaints.

- **Conversion Disorder:** this one happens when an individual shows physical symptoms that are the same as neurological disorder symptoms, although, in the real sense, they are not suffering from a neurological disorder. Symptoms include loss of hearing and vision, seizures, and paralysis. Generally, it comes as a result of trauma and affects an individual's movement and senses.

- **Pain Disorder:** pain disorder is characterized by pain in one or several body parts that keep on recurring with an unknown cause. It is diagnosed when a medical or other disorder cannot establish the cause of pain. Pain that caused distress with psychological factors playing a vital role at the beginning can also lead to its diagnosis depending on the amount and duration of such pain.

- **Hypochondriasis:** it occurs when minor symptoms and typical body signs are believed to be evidence of chronic illness, regardless of whether medical assessments and tests show otherwise. Physical symptoms can be either imagined or real.

- **Specified Somatic Symptoms:** the degree and threshold of these symptoms are below the criteria required to be diagnosed as somatoform disorder, but they include most of the symptoms. They include mild somatic symptoms disorder, illness anxiety, and brief illness anxiety disorder.

- **Unspecified Somatic Symptoms:** this applies to persons who have symptoms that show characteristics of somatic disorders but cannot be diagnosed as such because their degree and threshold is less than the established criteria for a somatoform disorder.

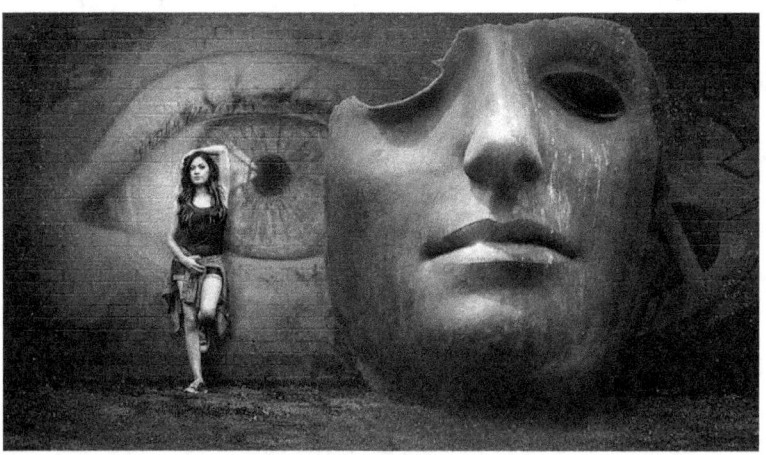

Symptoms Of Somatoform Disorders Include:

- Worrying persistently of possible sickness

- An impairment that is more significant form than what

is typical from medical circumstances.

- Interpreting familiar bodily sensations as severe physical sickness

- seeing symptoms as life-threatening or dire without medical facts or confirmation

- failure to have faith in medical treatment or assessment

Stress Disorders

Both are mental health conditions caused by witnessing or experiencing a terrifying event. Stress disorder can be looked at in two ways.

- **Post-Traumatic Stress Disorder (PTSD):** symptoms may appear suddenly or after sometime, get worse, and persist for months or years, and interfere with your life.

- **Acute Stress Disorder (ASD):** symptoms appear immediately after the traumatic events and last less than thirty days.

Signs Of Stress Disorders

Acute stress disorders begin almost immediately, after witnessing or going through the trauma usually within one month. A person temporarily finds it hard to adjust and cope, but they often, get better after a short period of good self-care. With post-traumatic stress disorder, symptoms tend to worsen. They last for long and take months or years and begin to interfere with a person's day-to-day functioning. Both ASD and PTSD share five broad categories of symptoms as follows:

- **Intrusion symptoms:** a person keeps on revisiting the traumatic event via dreams, memories, and flashbacks

- **Arousal symptoms:** the person feels on guard, and can quickly become startled, becomes irritable or aggressive either physically or verbally, has insomnia and other sleep disturbances and finds it difficult to concentrate.

- **Negative mood:** a pattern of low moods, negative thoughts, and sadness

- **Avoidance symptoms:** the person tends to avoid places, people, feelings, or thoughts associated with traumatic events

- **Dissociative symptoms:** characterized by an inability to remember episodes of the traumatic event, a lack of awareness of the surrounding and distorted sense of reality

Anxiety Disorders

Normal anxiety is healthy for achieving our goals and achievements. But when anxiety goes overboard and begins to interfere with our overall wellbeing and daily functioning, then it becomes a mental health condition that can lead to distress. When anxiety reaches such pathological levels, it is called an anxiety disorder. Here are some of the most prevalent types of anxiety disorders.

- **Panic disorders:** characterized by a feeling of random terror. One may also experience chest pains, strong irregular heartbeats, sweating, and a feeling of choking or having a heart attack.

- **Specific phobias:** extreme fear of particular situations or objects, including flights or heights.

- **Social anxiety:** also known as a social phobia: characterized by self-consciousness and overwhelming worry on social situations, fear of being judged, ridiculed, or embarrassed by others.

- **Generalized anxiety disorder:** a feeling of unrealistic and excessive worry accompanied by tension with no real cause.

Depression Disorders

These entail severe sadness that interferes with ones' daily activities and normal functioning. They include:

- Major depression, also known as a unipolar disorder.

- Persistent depression disorder

- Premenstrual dysphoric disorder

Symptoms Of Depression

- Sad, anxious and feelings of emptiness that persist and linger on

- Suicidal thought or attempts

- Body aches, headaches, cramps, and pains that rarely go away.

- Loss of interest in pleasurable things including sex

- Problems with digestion that worsen even with treatment

- feelings of worthlessness, helplessness and guilty

- restlessness and irritability

- being pessimistic and helpless

- trouble making decisions, concentrating and remembering details

- you may overeat or lose appetite completely

Social Psychology

Social psychology entails learning how actual, implied, or imagined presence of other people influences one's behaviors, feelings, and thoughts. In other words, it is focused on looking at how influence from others affects our actions, emotions, and thinking. The way a person perceives themselves relative to the surrounding world has a vital role in their beliefs, behavior, and the choices they make. The opinion of other people affects the way we view ourselves and our overall behavior.

There are significant research areas of social psychology as follows:

- **Attitude and attitude change:** this touches on attitudes, their development, and attitude changes. It is concerned with the ABCs of attitude which describes our feelings behavior and understanding

- **Violence and aggression:** this is more on trying to understand why people act aggressively and engage in violence. It looks at how social learning relates to sparking violent actions and behavior that tend to be aggressive.

- **Prosocial behavior:** this focuses on trying to understand why people help and cooperate with others, as well as why they don't.

- **Prejudice and discrimination:** this studies stereotypes, discrimination, and prejudice in social groups, and why these prejudices continue to exist even if there is evidence that contradicts them.

- **Self and social identity:** this is more on how we come to accept and appreciate ourselves and how our self-acceptance affects impact our relationships with others. It focuses on self-concept, self-esteem, self-awareness, and self-awareness, and how our inner self affects our outer person and social world.

- **Group behavior:** studies on why groups behave differently from individuals. Group behavior can be harmful and detrimental or positive and beneficial. Concepts in this area include group influence, group decision making, group dynamics, conflicts, leadership, and cooperation.

- **Social influence:** this focuses on the role of social influence of decision making and behavior. Concepts covered include the psychology of persuasion, conformity, obedience, and peer pressure.

- **Interpersonal relationships:** this studies social relationships and how to shape our feeling, thoughts, attitudes, and behavior. It looks at the importance of interpersonal relationships and how they affect us.

- **Social cognition:** it entails studying how social information can be applied after being processed and stored well.

Darwin's Theory of Evolution

Charles Darwin is well known in many countries across the world as the one who came up with the Theory of evolution. His Theory explains the continuous changes that happen within species from one generation to another, as well as the formation of new species due to environmental changes that affect the reproduction success of all individuals.

Darwin suggested that all species have a shared origin, change as time progresses, and new species are formed from existing ones. Each species continues to evolve with a unique set of traits or heritable characteristics that are different from the species of origin. These heritable differences accumulate gradually over a long period. As new species repeatedly split from their origin, they form a tree with the different level that connects all the living organisms to their origin. This change in which living things change their genetic features over generations enables them to evolve their abilities to adapt to their environment.

This Theory focuses on two aspects, namely, adaptation and natural selection. These two aspects shape how genes or alleles are inherited within a given population. Three inferences can be drawn for Darwin's five fundamental observations.

Darwin's observations

- All organisms have the fertility capability to increase the size of their population exponentially given that all the individuals born go on and reproduce again with success.

- Except for seasonal fluctuations, the size of the populations remains stable.

- Environmental resources like food or water are short in supply

- No two individuals are precisely the same in a population. Individuals extensively vary in characteristics that affect their reproduction and survival ability.

- Much of the difference in character can be inherited.

Explanation

- Species struggle to exist due to limited resources. That means only a small number of offspring will survive and successfully reproduce in each generation.

- A random process does not determine individuals who will survive to reproduce, but it depends on their genetic/hereditary constitution. Individuals with inherited characteristics that make them suitable to the environment they are living in may reproduce and have offspring other than the less adapted ones. By definition, this is called natural selection.

- As the population continues to evolve gradually through natural selection, individuals with favorable characteristics to survive will accumulate over the generations than those that are less suitable to survive and reproduce.

Individual's adaptation to the environment and their successful reproduction is differentiated through natural selection. Innate ability to adapt and survive is determined by unique suitable characteristics such as the pattern of behavior, anatomical structures, or physiological processes.

Natural Selection

If Darwin had just proposed them Theory of evolution and left it there, the chances are high that he would not be famous as he is today. What gets him into every textbook is because he went further and coined a formula known as "natural selection." The mechanism of natural selection aimed at logically explaining the evolution of the population. Populations underwent what Darwin referred to as "descent with modification," in a way that they become well adapted to their surroundings.

The idea of natural selection is anchored on some concrete observations.

- Traits can be inherited: characteristics are passed on from or inherited by the offspring from the parent. Thought Darwin was not aware of genes; he knew that was the case.

- Young ones get produced more than they can survive: individuals can produce more young ones than the environment can accommodate. That means, in each generation, the limited available resources will be competed for.

- There is a variation of heritable traits among offspring: in terms of features such as shape, size, color and other heritable traits, young ones in every generation will be somehow altered and show a slight difference from previous generations.

From these observations, Darwin came up with the following conclusions:

- Based on environmental conditions, such as the resources present and predators, some species will have hereditable features that will enable them to survive and reproduce. The species with desirable characteristics will leave more young ones in the next generation than others. This is because of the desirable traits that make it possible to survive and reproduce.

- Since the favorable characteristics can be inherited, and individual species with these features leave more young ones, these features will continue to be more prevalent from one generation to the next.

- The population of the species with these favorable features will become adapted to the environment over generations because of their consistent greater reproduction success.

This mechanism of natural selection helped Darwin explain his observations as he traveled. For instance, the finch had a shared origin, and it was possible and sensible to resemble each other. However, isolating groups of finches on different highlands for so many years would lead to the development of different species of finch on each highland. This is because of the various environmental factors which would have favored different heritable features like the length and the thickness of beaks for due to different food sources.

Natural Selection at Work

Take a population of mice with an inheritable variation of their fur color, such as tan versus black, moving into new surroundings which have many black rocks. In that new surroundings, mice eating hawks are prevalent, meaning that they can spot the tans more clearly than the blacks in that background of black rocks.

That means the tan mice will be eaten more than the black mice because their far color makes then vulnerable as they appear conspicuous in the new environment, while the back ones blend well against the black rocks and cannot be spotted with ease. At the end of it all, a large number of the tan mice will be consumed by the hawks, compared to a smaller number of black mice. In the end, the population of tans in the group that will survive is lower as compared to the starting population, while that of back ones will be larger.

The colorization of far is a feature that can be inherited from one generation to the next generation. That means, there will be a more significant number of the mice with black far in the group that will survive, hence more black offspring in the subsequent generation. With time, it means that the population will almost entirely be composed of blacks after several generations of natural selection.

Natural selection is environmentally depended: inherited superior genes are not favored by natural selection. It favors traits that are helpful in a particular environment. Desirable characteristics are beneficial in helping an individual for survival and reproduction, in a way that is effective than other organisms in that specific environment. Traits may work in a particular environment but fail in a different one.

Heritable variation forms the basis for natural selection: for the process of natural selection to commence, it needs some materials to start with. Heritable variation is, therefore, the material. There must be a variation on a feature that natural selection will work on. Such differences among the individuals have to be heritable.

Random mutations lead to heritable variation: random mutation is the originals source of new genes that produce new hereditary features. These changes in DNA sequences are passed on to offspring to make more variations.

The Importance of Evolution

Understanding evolution forms the basis of how we can find a solution to various problems that affect us.

- **In medicine:** Researchers have to understand the patterns of evolution of various organisms that cause different diseases so that they can stay one step ahead of these pathogenic diseases. Also, researchers have to study the history of how various disease-causing germs evolve so that they can gain knowledge of how to manage hereditary diseases.

- **Agriculture:** understanding the link between evolution and genetic variation enables farmers to enhance the potential of crops to fight diseases. Also following the evolution of pesticide resistance helps in devising methods of reducing crop damage by pests. In this case, understanding evolution can improve human life by securing the world's food supply.

- **Conservation:** knowledge of evolutions helps us to conserve endangered species. Having an awareness of the link between the size of the population and how the genes vary, we can realize when a population is facing the danger of extermination. Hatcheries' artificial selection can affect the density of the population in the wild when such hatchery fish are let out. Conservationists can make better decisions on where to focus their effort using the knowledge of polygenetic with an eye on biodiversity.

- **Drug development:** new drugs have to be tested for their usability by humans, but they cannot be given directly to humans before a variety of safety factors have been established. Knowledge of evolution reminds us that we have a common origin with other animals like macaques or the dog. Drugs are therefore piloted on the first, before being distributed for use by humans. The practical application of evolution can help pharmaceutical companies save billions of dollars during this process.

- **Antibiotic resistance:** once, penicillin used to work miracles in human health. Today professionals are waking to the reality of a host of diseases that have evolved resistance to antibiotics. The fact that organisms can develop resistance to medicines is a classic example of natural selection. Antibiotics are usually given to patients with infections from a diverse population of bacteria. These antibiotics have the potential to wipe out all the bacteria. But sometimes when they feel better, they stop using the antibiotics without finishing the dosage. That means bacteria that are most resistant to the antibiotics will be left behind. These surviving bacteria become a nucleus of a new and more resilient population. Such knowledge of bacterial evolution is vital to secure public health.

Evolution Today

Today we witness evolution in almost every area of our lives. Evolution is taking place in medicine, agriculture, and technology. Technology is bringing tremendous changes in nearly every field, making life easier with ease to solve complex problems. Let's look at the changes which are taking place in nature and technology.

Examples of Evolution in Nature

- Insecticide resistance: mosquitoes are becoming resistant to various insecticides. As a result of an insect being exposed to such chemicals for long, specific genetic changes occur in the insect, and it mutates to develop such resistance.

- Pesticide resistance: some crop pathogens have become resistant to pesticides. Regular use of a similar class of chemicals to prevent pest leads to mutation of the genes. Hence the resistance.

- Antibiotics resistance: some bacteria are developing resistance to drugs. Some of the drugs such as penicillin which used to work a miracle in wiping out a variety of bacterial resistance are no longer effective.

- Lactose intolerance in humans: according to the scientist, nine percent of humans genes are evolving at the moment. These are genes in sexual reproduction, sensory perception, and immune system. An example of natural selection can be seen in the fact that humans are the only species that doesn't become intolerant to lactose.

- Sickle hemoglobin gene: this gene mutation happened in some areas of Africa due to exposure to malaria. Because of the ongoing exposure to malaria in successive generations, this mutation has made them more resistant to malaria.

- Interaction between crabs and mussels: blue mussels

have been observed to thicken their shells when the sense or spot crabs. This behavior is typical in mussels in Asian shores where there are endemic crabs.

- Rat snake: rat snakes live in the eastern half of the United States, and their skin colorization has been observed to be green, orange, yellow, or black depending on their environment.

Evolution Examples in Technology

- The size of computers has decreased from big sizes that filled an entire room to computer screens as small as a watch face

- Screens of televisions have exponentially increased from small 12-inch screens to current screens that are the size of an entire room

- The mobile industry has experienced tremendous changes. The size of cell phones has changed over the years from large sizes that were the size of a suitcase, to very small sizes that fit in one's hearing. Today, a cell phone screen is like a complete computer screen with so many features.

Chapter 6: Psychological Functionalist

Structuralism is a term used to describe the school of psychology, which was the first to emerge. It focused on breaking down the processes of the mind into foundational components to form the basis for the study. To understand the basics of these components of consciousness, leaners used a method of study called introspection.

Wilhelm Wundt founded the first psychology lab and is associated with this school of psychology. This school of thought was criticized because the methods used to study the mind's structure were believed to be so objective. The use of introspection produced unreliable results. It was concerned with internal behavior, which cannot be observed directly or measured accurately.

That is not to means that structuralism was insignificant. It was the first primary school in psychology, and this structuralism school contributed to the development of experimental psychology.

Functionalism was formed to counter structuralism and was primarily impacted by the works of William James, together with the theory of evolution, which was first proposed by Charles Darwin. These functionalists strived to study and explain the processes of the mind accurately and systematically.

Instead of looking at consciousness elements, functionalist concentrated on the intent of behavior and consciousness. They too stressed individual differences, which had a profound effect on education. Functionalism was an essential influence on psychology. It led to the development of applied psychology and behaviorism. It also impacted on education following the belief of Dewey that a child should learn when they reached developmental preparedness. Well, known functionalists are people like William James and Harvey Carr.

Functionalism was famously criticized by Wundt, who rubbished it as beautify literature with no basis in psychology.

Structure Versus Physiology

Structure

This is the scientific study of the body's structures. Some of our body structures are very tiny, and one has to use a microscope to observe and analyze them. Other structures are readily visible can be measured, weighted, and manipulated. Structure or anatomy originates from the Greek root that means to cut apart. At first human structures were understood by observing the external body parts and watching the wounds of injured soldiers and other bodily injuries.

With time, physicians began to dissect dead bodies to study internal parts and increase their knowledge. Such internal structures are cut apart after the body has been dissected, to be observed separately to determine their relationships to one another and determine their physical characteristics. Today this dissecting method is still used in medical schools, pathology labs, and anatomy courses. However, several imaging techniques have been developed to aid in the observation of structures in living people. They help in visualizing structures such as a cancerous tumor or fractured bones inside the body. Anatomy or structure has the following areas of specialization:

- Gross anatomy: this entails the study of larger body structures, which are visible without using any magnification aid. It is also known as macroscopic anatomy. Macro means large.

- Microscopic anatomy: micro means small. It involves

the study of tiny body statures that can only be seen or observed with any of the magnification instruments such as a microscope. It consists of the study of cells which is called cytology, and the study of tissues which is referred to as histology.

There are two general approaches that anatomists use to study body structure.

- Regional anatomy: this is the learning of how structures in a specific body structure, such as the abdomen, are interrelated. Regional anatomy helps us to understand and appreciate how different body part such as blood vessels, muscles, nerves, and other structures interrelate and work together to serve a particular region of the body.

- Systemic anatomy: this focuses on studying structures that make up a discrete body system. Such a structure usually works together to perform a specific body function. For instance, a systemic study of the muscular system takes into consideration all the body's skeletal muscles.

Physiology

Unlike structure, physiology is about how these body structures function. It focuses on the physics and the chemistry of the body structures and the different ways in which they work together to aid life functions. Much of the body physiology centers on homeostasis. Homeostasis is a steady-state of internal conditions maintained by the body. Just like structure, physiology entails observing with naked eyes, use of magnification devices such as the microscope, measurement, and manipulation. However, physiology has currently advanced and largely depends on keenly designed experiments in the laboratory. These experiments aid in revealing the functions of various body structures along with the chemical compounds present in the human body.

Just like in the case of structure, physiology has various fields of specialization. For instance, neurophysiology involves the study of the human brain. They work together to achieve complex and diverse functions such as thinking, vision, and movement. Physiology may work form:

- Organ level: for example, exploring the work of the different brain parts.

- Molecular-level: for example, exploring how electromagnetic signals travel along nerves.

Form and function are closely related. The study of structure and physiology makes more sense if the form of the structures and their functions are continually related. It can be frustrating to try to understand a body structure without knowledge of the physiology that the structure supports. For example, think of a situation where you are trying to appreciate how bones are uniquely arranged in your hand without any concept of how the hand functions. First by observing how you use your hand to manipulate different devices such as how you hold a pen and operate a cell phone, makes it easy for you to appreciate while the thumb is aligned in opposition to the other four fingers. Hence, your hand becomes a structure that fulfills the physiology of grasping objects.

Thus, structure or anatomy is a scientific study that helps us to understand the body structures. Physiology, on the other hand, explains how these body structures work together to maintain life. It focuses on the physics and the chemistry behind these body structures. It is an uphill task to study structure without the concept or knowledge of function. Typically, structure and physiology or form and functions are considered together because they are closely related, and you cannot understand one without the other.

The Mind as the Brain's Software

The relationship between the mind and the brain is a complex one, and sometimes we tend to assume that the brain and the mind are the same. Take an example where you are told to use one of your fingers to point to your brain, and then told to use the same finger to point to your mind. The chances are that your figure will remain positioned where it was. You will be unable to figure out the difference between the locations of your mind separate from your brain. Due to the complicated relationship between the mind and the brain, these two words are used interchangeably in our cultures.

That notwithstanding, the brain and the mind are not the same. They refer to separate but often overlapping, concepts. The brain is a physical part of the body that is visible and tangible. The mind, on the other hand, transcendent invisible or the unseen metaphysical world of thought, imagination, belief, feeling and attitude. The brain forms the body organ that is associated with the mind, while the mind cannot be limited to the brain, because the mind's intelligence is not limited to the brain cells, but permeates every other part and organ of the body. The mind is independent of the brain and has immense potential over all the systems of the body. It is the mind that gives humans control over the working of their brains.

The relationship between the mind and the brain can be thought to be the same as the relationship between computer hardware and software. A computer cannot perform its functions without the hardware. Software is required so that the hardware can run. Without the software, the hardware becomes useless; it can't perform its functions. What the hardware does is determined by the software, and the hardware performs as good as the software installed in it. But without the hardware, however powerful the software is, it remains useless.

The brain acts as hardware while the mind acts as a software. Either cannot perform without the other. But in reality, the complicated relationship between the brain and the mind is far much complex than just a computer and computer program.

The brain is a part of the body organs while the mind is not. The brain is the body organ that houses the mind. It contains electronic impulses that create thoughts. The brain is used to transmit impulses, coordinate movement, and the whole-body organism. But the mind is used to think to tell the brain what to do. With the mind, you can muse at what transpired in the past, what will happen in the future and what has just happened now.

The brain can be said to be the manifestation of what takes place in the brain such as thoughts, memory, imagination perceptions and attitudes. The mind is associated with the thought process of reason and logic. The mind makes us conscious and aware. The mind controls what we do, and makes us know how to do it and why we are doing it. The mind is the ability to understand processes. An animal can interpret their environment, but they cannot understand it. Humans have an understanding of the happenings around them and can adapt or make some changes to their environment.

The mind is the logic that makes humans solve the complex logical problem, differentiating them from other living things. It is the mind that gives us the power to analyze complex situations and use logic to understand things differently from what they may see. We use the mind to come up with solutions to different problems that we face. Though we are unable to see in the ultraviolet range with our naked eyes, we use the mind to develop devices to enable us to see. We can use our minds to build real knowledge and give away our superstitious ways by making observation and experiment with reality. We use our minds to make new scientific discovering by developing sophisticated devices through the logic power of the mind.

Speaking, the relationship between the mind the brain is the most complex and challenging one. By thinking of the mind as the software of the mind, we draw a lot of insight into understanding this complex and almost overlapping concept. The brain is a powerful organ, and the mind is the neural software that resides in it, enabling it to accomplish complex processes and functionalities. Neither can function without the other.

The Nervous System

It is composed of nerves and cells. These cells, plus the nerves, are joined together in a complex network. They carry impulses to the other parts of the body and organs. It consists of the center together with the peripheral system. The center has the brain together with the spinal cord. The peripheral has automatic and somatic systems.

The Central Nervous System (CNS)

The brain and the spinal cord are part of it. It is shaped like a mushroom, weighs less than 1.5 kgs and found inside the skull. It has supporting cells and nerve cells, namely glia and neurons, respectively.

In the brain, there is some matter that is tasked with performing two different functions. One of them has neuroglia as well as the cell bodies and works to store messages after receiving them, and it is known as the grey matter. The other type of matter woks to carry messages and information the grey matter or from it. This has nerve fibers, as well as axons which make it possible to accomplish the work of carrying impulses, and it is known as the grey matter.

Spinal Cord

- It is relatively long and structured like a tube and makes an extension of the brain. It is approximately 45 centimeters and weighs around 40g. It is housed inside the backbone, specifically the vertebral column and divided further into segments which are 31 in member.

- Every segment has one pair of nerves extending from it. Motor/ sensory never are also part of the cord.

Parts of the Brain

- **Brain stem:** This has been estimated to around one inch in length, and its location lies between the other two parts. One of these parts is called the pons, while the other part is called the spinal cord. The medulla oblongata is the other name of the brain stem.

- **Diencephalon:** can also know as to as the forebrain stem and is known to consist of the hypothalamus and the thalamus. Sensory impulses, as well as other types of impulses, come to coalesce at the thalamus, while they hypothalamus will just form a small part if the diencephalon.

- **Midbrain:** provides the pathways for conducting to/from the lower and other centers that are higher in the brain.

- **Pons:** contains conducting paths to/from the higher brain centers and the medulla. It is the pathway to higher structures.

- **The cerebrum:** is anchored on the brain stem forming the base of the brain and has hemispheres that a known to be two in number. The again have lobes which total to four in number. They are frontal, occipital, parietal, and temporal. The wok of the hemispheres is for each to regulate body activates on the side opposite side of its location.

- **The cerebellum:** is situated below and behind the cerebrum.

- **Meninges:** are the three membranes or layers that protect the cord and the brain. They are arranged in layers as external, middle, and the inner membranes are namely Dura mater, arachnoid, and the pia matter respectively. They act as barriers against microorganisms and bacteria, and they work to protect the cord and the brain.

- **Cerebrospinal Fluid (CSF):** flows around the cord and brain, nourishing them as well as protecting them.

- **Neurons:** are cells that are specialized for conduction and form a fundamental part of the brain and the cord. Its work is to receive and carry messages and information in the form of impulses or electrochemical. It consists of axons, dendrites, and cell bodies, which help in carrying impulses to different body parts and organs. The cell body has a nucleus and acts as the control center. The axon is long and thin, working to carry messages out of the cell body to other neurons or tissues. In the motor neuron, the dendrite has several highly branched extensions to form a cable-like network. In the sensory neuron, it is made of along dendrite. The dendrite carries impulses into the cell body.

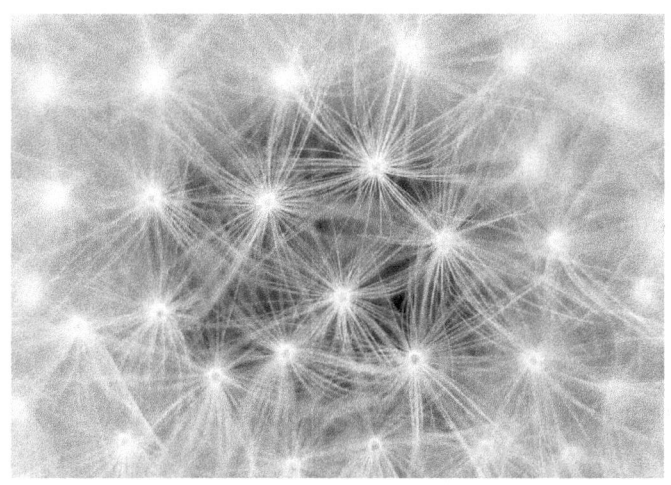

Peripheral Nervous System

This system encompasses the automatic and somatic systems. The somatic contains nerves that pick sensory messages or sensations from organs that are far from the brain, such as the arms or legs and takes them to the brain. It also contains motor nerve fibers coming from the brain that carry information to the skeletal muscles for action. The automatic encompasses enteric, sympathetic and the parasympathetic systems. They work together to control body activities such as breathing, heartbeat, and digestion, which cannot be controlled consciously by humans.

The Endocrine System

The endocrine system encompasses bodily glands that make various chemicals and hormones for helping cells to communicate with each other. These hormones are responsible for the functioning of cells, organs, and the body.

A gland is a small organ responsible for producing hormones that aid the body in performing a particular function. They release these chemicals into the blood, which takes them to the desired organs.

Functions of the Endocrine System

- Makes hormones responsible for performing different functions in the body.

- It controls how different hormones will be released in the body

- It releases the necessary chemical into the bloodstream

Parts of the Endocrine System

It encompasses all the different glands in the body. Some are in the brain, such as the hypothalamus, pineal gland, and pituitary. At the neck, we have parathyroid and thyroid glands. At the pelvic region, we have testes and the ovaries. The adrenal glands are situated on kidneys. The pancreas is located in the stomach area while the thymus is between the lungs.

- **Hypothalamus:** it is responsible for linking the endocrine to the nervous system. It tells the pituitary gland when to commence the production of different bodily chemicals and hormones.

- **The pituitary gland:** is the fundamental gland in this system. It receives the brains that give signals to this gland, which then communicates to the rest of the glands in the body on what to do, depending on the nature of the information given. It also makes important hormones that are responsible for growth like prolactin and luteinizing hormone. Prolactin aids in milk production during breastfeeding, while luteinizing controls testosterone in males and estrogen in the female

- **Thyroid gland:** It makes thyroid hormone, which regulates metabolism. If it fails to produce enough and condition called hypothyroidism, the body metabolism slows down, and everything begins to happen in a slow manner. This may lead to a slow heart rate, weight gain, or get constipated. In the case of hyperthyroidism, where it makes too much hormone, everything speeds up. The heart races, you may lose weight or experience diarrhea.

- **Pineal gland:** produces melatonin chemical that prepares the body for sleep

- **Adrenals glands:** they are responsible for generating the hormones that help us escape danger. They also produce hormones that influence metabolism and sexual functions.

- **Parathyroid glands:** these are little glands situated at the backside of the thyroid. They are four in number, and they are responsible for the health of the bones. They regulate the level of phosphorus and calcium.

- **Pancreas:** works in both the digestive and the endocrine systems. It releases enzymes that help in the breakdown of food. It helps in maintaining blood sugar by releasing insulin and glycogen into the bloodstream.

- **Thymus gland:** this gland is responsible for making white blood cells that fight infections. These blood cells are called T-lymphocytes. They are vital in developing the immune system of a child. After puberty, the thymus begins to vanish.

- **Ovaries:** they are found in women and are tasked with the production of progesterone and estrogen. They are responsible for the growth of breasts during puberty. They also control the menstrual cycle and maintaining pregnancy.

- **Testes:** they are found in males and are responsible for producing testosterone. It is responsible for the growth of hair during puberty aids in enlarging the penis and production of sperms.

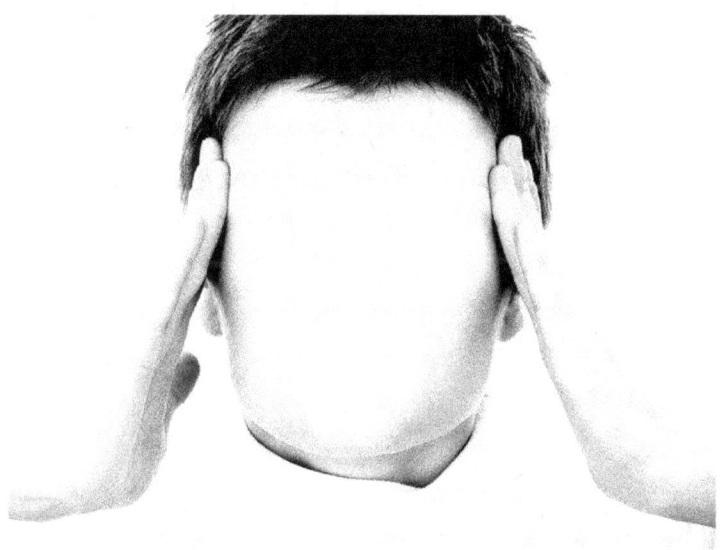

Chapter 7: Brief Guide to Further Issues and Applications

Human behavior and the brain is tracked and studied via psychology. To obtain information on the cognitive functions the mind undergoes a series of tests and procedures that help psychologists have an understanding. Psychological knowledge can be split into a series of disciplines that help advance and learn how the mind is receptive or functions under different circumstances. Whenever the brain is faced with a situation it acts by controlling the behavior, thoughts, etc. The brain is be divided into hemispheres which assist psychologist to understand cognitive behavior. Discussed are some of the applications of psychology and how we relate to either directly or indirectly.

Mindset Psychology

There are factors that influence how we think and perceive what surrounds us. Mindset, therefore, is the belief in us that directs how we take care of situations. These beliefs draw lines between people since they are not homogenized. People are different so are their beliefs. Mindsets can be categorized into two broad categories; growth mindset and fixed mindset. With a growth mindset, there is a window of change in the way the mind sees situations. In a fixed mindset, we so much entrust our skills, experiences, talents, intelligence, etc.

A growth mindset requires an open mind. With a growth mindset, the idea is to be in harmony with life-threatening situations that might have been experienced, struggles, setbacks, etc. To fuse up with these situations and toughen up one requires to realize what potential they hold and what can come out of them. Since it is a growth mindset, the time has to be invested for it to pay off. The time is invested in making the mind see things it had never thought via another channel and avenue. Focus is pointed at the individual developing more skills and abilities. With more consistency, the ideas and skills are recorded in the brain and thereafter the brain no longer attacks situations via the same avenue used earlier.

Mindsets can be changed by the interest of and individual to learn or drop behavior that is fixed. It is not something that can change instantly, the brain has to get challenged so that it can accept the new beliefs. It has been proven that speaking highly of one's intelligence will squash their motivation and also brings about a decline in the performance. Psychological advice to help people with fixed mindsets to love challenges since they are part of life. Learning from our mistakes helps the mind change the mindset. To achieve a complete change in mindset one has to accept whatever life brings at us but one should also consider. Being born with top-notch abilities does not mean one is special. Similar abilities can be gained by someone who is neither talented or gifted but he or she fights to learn the skill and perfect it.

Mindset is very important in life; it will determine who it is that you will interact with and who you won't. People prefer people with a growth mindset to those of a fixed mindset. To be in a position that you can understand a person your mindset has to accommodate some of the new concepts. A fixed mindset will end up turning down an even better option that would be of help. Psychologists try to campaign for the growth mindset which is time-sensitive and absorbing new methodologies. I believe someone with a mindset that is growing and that is able to add more information to itself is a favored individual. The mind happens to be the one organ that has been of interest to human and they never understand it fully.

The Active Mind

An active mind is the section of the mind that acts on sensory impulses received and provides a new meaning to them. The mind is however believed to be preconditioned. This is true to a point but has remained under challenge with new knowledge emerging and more experiments. An active mind is able to turn sensory impulses into experiences that are stored and processed. They help us be who we are eventually. Bandura (1963) concedes some habits make who we are since they were acquired via direct training and perhaps conditioning. Patterns of personality are closely linked to our parents or those that molded our early age development. this displays the power of an active mind.

Bandura (1963) uses an example of punishment as a form of instilling discipline while providing punishment the active art of the mind collects the reason for the punishment and records. After recording it, it becomes rare of a repeat of the same due to the fact that the punishment help shaped behavior. Via training the active mind is able to hold information and process it hence creating an experience. Bandura (1989) worked on the social cognitive theory. Modeling is actively stimulating the active mind. Modeling furthermore can assist us to develop cognitive abilities, morality, judgment, etc. With active mind ideas are necessarily not enough to create an experience that displays how we respond. We respond differently depending on our conditioned and trained abilities. The active mind is responsible for the application of entirely different things along our life paths.

Children are able to learn linguistics entirely by being close to the parents or guardians who are actively talking. The active mind takes on the challenge and helps develop the linguistic area of kids. An active mind can be accessed through training therefore for these kids to gain more skills and experience the parents can promote this by bringing onboard new elements. Active learning can be applied in more areas like learning to ride a bicycle etc.

We can learn almost everything in this world that is there to be learned. With an active mind, the sensory stimulant is active and records all that happens hence creating a window that helps us improve on self. When we learn new techniques especially under training or interest it sticks and makes us better at that which we thought would never be good at. It is also advice able to avoid instilling fear in a child in his or her learning process. The active mind can be influenced by fear leading to the poor recording of methodologies learned.

Gentle handling of situations will enhance active mind learning. People are different though; some prefer forceful learning while others require a slow learning process for the active mind to grab the information and make it part of someone. The active mind is so receptive and powerful.

Children, for instance, will learn how to walk and talk from their parents. The active mind of a kid should be recorded as the most attentive and active.

Nutritional psychology

It is the psychological study of the cognitive choices on meals. These decisions have a substantial influence on the overall health, psychological capacity, and nutrition. With this field, psychologists try to uncover and establish any links that exist between the mental health of an individual with nutritional behavior. Our feeding habits tell a lot, how fast, or slow we eat, what we eat and how frequent are just a few guidelines on feeding habits. How we live and it contributes so much to our mental and overall health.

Our diets help us perform our daily tasks with ease. Psychologists in the field would advise students to invest in diets that will boost their memory and the overall activity of the brain. Foods that boost the activity of the brain help us think better and make sound decisions. The brain happens to be one of the most important and fragile body organs. If it is well maintained via healthy feeding and living it can do orders.

Nutrition psychology tries to identify cures to issues like stress that can also be caused by nutritional negligence. Nutrients are fuels of this body hence negligence will only lead to complications. Nutritional psychology has the following applications;

Food Technology

In most countries, food packaged has some laws that require them to label the containers with information about the product. The labels show ingredients, amount and some even go as far as entailing the health advantages of the product. Nutritional psychologists engage in research and try to discover the influence these labels have on the consumers of the products. Research reveals that most consumers have no eye for the label hence continued cases of lifestyle diseases. Advice is that one should read the labels to be diet conscious and also be able to analyze the ingredients.

Marketing

Marketing means more sales hence more profits and production. Young people are mostly the target of this food marketing strategies since the adults don't easily fall into the trap. Young consumers are easily impressed by these advertisements. With new packaging of the foodstuff and strong marketing moves, obesity sets in. it becomes the work of nutritional psychologists to fight and regulate the advertisements on food and beverages.

FAD Diets

Nutrition psychologists are interested in how we eat and the exercise we also take. Fad diets are a quick fix to issues of weight loss, some have other health advantages. This may be true but the ingredients are capable of bringing about fatal if not serious problems. Nutritional psychologists help in providing the information and statics of the dietary. They also delve into the fad diets hence try to establish the efficacy of the drug.

Food Technology

Nutritional psychologists are also involved in the studies of what people tell about food evolutionary. People prefer organic food to technologically modified. Nutritionally the technology modified food is more fortified and nutritious. People only feel safe with organic food since the genetically modified food is a whole new line of foodstuff.

What we eat tells more of our pockets and abilities. We eat what we can afford. Many consumers are not concerned with the ingredients as long as it is sweet or serves the purpose of filling their belies and providing fuel for performing daily tasks. When we have a lot of brain activity, maybe while studying or thinking excessively, the brain requires nutrition and these are obtained from the body. Nutrition to be taken also depends on the richness of the nutrients i.e. the nutrient value.

Motivation and goals

Motivation involves factors that combine to harness and activate a behavior. This behavior is goal-oriented. Forces are in place that fuels our motives. Motives are the reasons we do what we do, they answer the question 'why' of certain behavior. Motivation requires three components. First is activation which is the decision that sets a behavior on its own course. Secondly, we have persistence which is the continued activities of effort to go on. The energy to continue with the decision no matter the obstacles ahead or circumstances. Thirdly, is intensity, grinding on and on to pursue what you set ahead. With goals these three principles matter. Motivations can either be extrinsic or intrinsic. Extrinsic motivations arise from the surrounding of an individual like gifts, cash, commendations, etc. Intrinsic motivations arise from deep within the individual as satisfaction or gratification.

Motivation can also be described via some theories put forward. The instinct theory states that habits are motivated by instincts. These are believed to be inborn and fixed and are very important for and organisms' survival. The theory of drives and needs, on the other hand, stipulates that our doings and habits are influenced and motivated by biology. There exists a biological need for some basic components of life like water, food, and sleep. We, therefore, get powered up to meet these needs and survive. The arousal levels theory puts it out that people engage in habits that help them have an optimal level of arousal. Those with low arousal find relaxing activities fine by them while those on a higher dose of arousal engage in thrilling activities that require quite some energy from them.

Goals are the final achievements of our hard work. Goals associated with school work mostly require intrinsic motivation. Passion is personal and therefore passionate students tend to show interest in their courses of choice all the way till they complete studies. It doesn't stop there, they continue till they have fulfillment in their hearts, that's when they feel that their goals are met.

Goals attained give a feeling of relief especially if the path to attaining the goal was no joke. Accomplished goals stimulate our brains and it doesn't stop there. We plan more and more goals and we feel happy when we accomplish one bone. We also provide ourselves with motivation aspects to help us achieve this dream. Faded dreams are hard to bring them up to speed and require patience and more understanding. The feeling of hitting a target set after a lot of tiling and almost giving up is overwhelming.

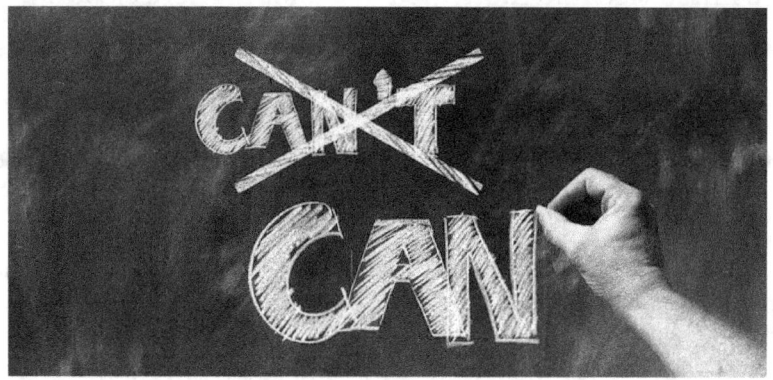

Optimism

Over time it has been confirmed that optimism is related to many positive life outcomes. The optimist has a better life. They have health advantages hanging on them. Optimists have a low risk of depression, they also have a lofty life expectancy, better and perfect mental health, general body wellness. Optimists are not realistic. Psychologists try to find out the survival tactics with the optimists. They are positive and fascinating with less of health conditions due to their lifestyle. Optimism reveals there is more good to live than bad.

Optimists have better strategies for coping with life quietly and effectively. They also practice better health habits. Optimism in high doses may lead to adversely risky habits while too much pessimism makes life unbearable.

Being optimistic helps one evade or face certain life situations with so much courage and positivity. Psychologically, optimists have this trait as a way of survival and also come up with other individuals. Psychologists that study the brain functionality believe that being a pessimist or an optimist depends on the hemisphere of the brain that is put to use mostly. Optimists have more physiological activity on their left hemispheres while their counterparts use the right hemisphere. Furthermore, optimists have high self-esteem, cheerful mood and they focus on wellness and the positive side of anything. The left hemisphere of the brain is responsible for handling stimuli and it is also attenuated towards the positives.

The left hemisphere radiates positivity. But we need both hemispheres of the brain. They work together and help create an impression of life. They come together and help mediate how we perceive the world and deal with it too. The optimist sees the world from an eye of less struggle and more perspiration.

Being optimist requires no license, though some people never bring down their egos so that issues can be resolved. Optimism brings better options that harm. The brain feels at peace and hence with that peace of mind, the optimists are able to focus. When there are some stirring issues both optimists and pessimists share the issue and try the find a way around it or just through it. Optimists rarely give up and talk ill of something no matter how grey it is.

Physical Exercise and Psychology

Physical exercises are so important to human beings. With physical exercises our bodies become fit and we experience more relaxation afterward. Doing exercises counteracts the effects of bad feeding habits and a lifestyle that is unhealthy. Therapists advise their patients to take good care of their bodies and do more exercise. Some exercises are so intense and hence such is only suitable for sports personnel and athletes. Exercises help treat lifestyle illnesses like hypertension and diabetes.

Sport and exercise psychology are disciplines that engage in scientific principles of exercise and sports. They try to understand and also find out the psychological factors that come linked to exercising ability and sports. With the knowledge obtained from these studies, sports psychologists advice trainers of athletes and sports persons on the best exercises that will yield more performance. For athletes and sportspeople, it is not just about fitness but ultimate performance is of key importance.

Exercise psychology also involves studies on how participation in physical exercises can add value to us. Actually, it has been discovered that frequent exercises add some years to our life span by boosting our wellness and health. Psychological development is also affected by the amount of time and energy we put into physical exercises. Engaging in exercises will help enhance our moods even shorter sessions of a physical exercise can have a great deal on our moods. Exercises, however, do not only mend our moods. They can also be used to treat panic disorders. When we find ourselves in compromised situations, the brain receives the information via neurons and processes it quick. The brain will stimulate the release of some of the body chemicals hormones. These hormones respond and cause a series of reactions that will lead to sweating, dizziness, etc.

Exercises make us also feel good about ourselves by improving our self-esteem. Accomplishing smaller milestones gives us some pride which translates to general happiness. The body image also can use some physical exercises and reshape it to a fit and attractive body. Depression is a situation that can be handled quite well with a dose of physical exercises daily as prescribed by the therapists or psychologists. In 3-4 weeks of continued physical exercises, depression is reduced and the individual feel good about themselves. Instances of depression are greatly reduced.

Neurotransmitters are freshened up and so is the body when we engage in physical exercises. Blood flow is increased due to the urgent requirement of nutrients to muscles and oxygen. With blood rushing via our veins during the exercise, the brain is accessed by the rushing blood and oxygen supply is boosted so the brain freshens up in the process. With patients of cholesterol disorders doing exercises is not an option rather a recommendation.

Athletes and sportsmen enjoy the fruits of sport psychology. It helps them improve on their performance and also help in their life by strengthening their bodies for more stress that they are likely to get exposed to as an occupational hazard. In case of accidents, the psychologists are important in advice and counseling.

Chapter 8: Positive Psychology of Time

In the world today, time has been referred to as a scarce resource which then requires deeper psychological revelation in order to determine the positivity of time. This is because it carries a lot of attributes. The academic sphere has been a major one when it comes to the consideration of time as a utility. We all have appreciated the scarcity of time. One day you are around, the next time you are not even in existence. Time has proven over and over of its scarcity. It is more than often that you would hear an academism referring to time as gold. We all have twenty-four hours a day to do whatever we desire and when this time lapses, all we can do is move on to the next day. When you compare time with money, you will find that time surpasses all resources. Time as a resource has always regained its value due to its scarcity. We have no control over time and because of this, you will find that it keeps escaping our mind. Most of the time we experience the feeling like instead of being in charge of our own time it is the one that is driving us crazy.

Positive psychology, on the other hand, entails how we best percept our lives. When we look at our lives in the best way possible that which makes it worth living then this is what is known as positive psychology. Life often throws around various obstacles that make it hard to live a smooth life. When we encounter various challenges, we learn from them and thus we can never be torn down by such events. Challenges give us another shot at life and enable us to have different perspectives about life. This is what makes life worth living. Imagine a life that is devoid of challenges and is almost as smooth as a tarmac road. In a nutshell, positive psychology is a study that focuses on the strengths of an individual rather than the weaknesses.

This chapter focuses on combining the scarcity of time as a factor and the positive psychology of individuals. When your psychology is influenced positively, you tend to dwell with positive thoughts, ones that uplift you and do not pull you down. When this happens, your mood is said to be always elevated. Positivism can be closely linked to optimism. An optimist is an individual who focuses all his or her attention on the events that will make him or her elevate his or her spirits. When you are in thoughts about what makes you feel happy, the brain releases chemicals known as endorphins that help a great deal in channeling the same feeling throughout the body. Research has it that people who are happy tend to live longer lives than those who drown themselves in sorrows all the time.

Time management, on the other hand, focuses on how best you can use your time in order to achieve the maximum out of it.

This entails engaging in a number of exercises that will see to it you manage your time properly. When we manage time properly, we are in a position to boost our productivity. When our productivity is enhanced, we make the most out of our lives. When we focus on how time enhances our productivity through time management, we focus wholly on how our well-being can be improved through time management. Research has it that when we engage all aspects of our life positively, we tend to benefit even more. Take for instance when accord time the respect it deserves and through positive psychology, we engage in the correct activities at the correct time, we will find that life turns out to be positive for us.

In order to accord time, the necessary attention, it requires, first you have to assume a positive attitude. One that you tell yourself time is there as a factor and the perception you accord it is how it is going to function to your advantage. When talking about creating time, one may think of it as the simplest of issues. How easy is it to free up some time in order to take up a task. However, time goes beyond freeing up some space in order to take up another task. As human beings, we have the habit of over-estimating the amount of time we accord to wok. Here we visualize that the time we have devoted to work is overwhelming. We do not want to restrict our free time and thus we tend to look down upon the time we have as free.

When we tend to think about how much time free time we have at our disposal in a week, many people may actually narrow it down to less than twenty hours. When you look at it in-depth, this is actually half of what we have. When we want to have a candid view of how time affects our lives, we tend to focus too much on what pushes us through boredom. In a bid to understand what eats up our time we tend to encounter various factors that are not of relative importance to ourselves. Channeling your time into positive thinking will see to it that you are a productive way more than you were before.

As human beings, we fail when we engage in various activities in order to satisfy our quotient of hobbies. For instance, you will find an individual who is playing rugby at the same time doing swimming at the same time going for mountain climbing and at the same time engaging in sky diving. Mostly when we achieve more, it is often as a result of straining time and over-exploitation of this resource. In order to use time in a manner that is fulfilling to ourselves, we ought to look at time in a manner that suggests we have keen decoding of time and its inner meaning. The psychology of time, for instance, is a factor that we ought to decode in a bid to secure ourselves within the restrictions of timelines. The psychology of time entails:

Perspective of Time

This refers to the actual visual imagination that you accord to time when you look around yourself. How you perceive time will best determine how you will manipulate it to your advantage. Time occurs in various tenses which include the present, future, and past not necessarily in seriatim. These tenses manifesting themselves in your life in ways that you cannot imagine. Take for instance an issue in the past that could be haunting you to the present. In order to secure your future, you need a stable job. In a nutshell, time perspective is the basis upon which we relay our thoughts in order to make decisions. Could it be the present, the past or the future? Time perspective goes beyond the three facets aforementioned in order to encompass five other facets. The facets include:

Future-Oriented People

These are individuals whose biggest focus is on the events that will happen in the future. Talk about perfectionists, these are your type of people. They will maintain a perfect record in a bid to secure a chance in the future. They are relentless in their way of doing things in that they do not give up quickly. These types of people are keen analysts who tend to evaluate the dangers of an event even before its occurrence. They have the perception that in order to enjoy in the future, you have to commit yourself to some extent in the present. They view enjoyment in the present as short term. With this kind of perception about time, this kind of person is often successful n life than others.

Present Hedonistic Individual

This is an individual who tends to live in the moment. These types of people have a kind of inborn hype that tends to make them live in the moment. Most of the time they would rather get results now than later. To them, consequences are a matter of now and then. Most of these people tend to be addicts since they easily give in to various temptations. Take for instance impulse buyers, drug addicts, and alcoholics. Most of these people are often failures due to their mistaken perception of time. They would accord very little time to matters that require substantial amounts of reasoning and contemplations.

Present Fatalistic Individuals

These people just as the above mention live in the present and have the tendency to act on impulse. Their impulse is however directed towards the feeling of turmoil and disassociation. These people live a lonely life since they have the belief that outside forces tend to affect one's life. Owing to this, they will lock everyone out in a bid to secure self-security. Most of these individuals do not associate properly with others. This is because they have a restricted personality. These people spend most of their time thinking about their emotions. The average performers and most of them above average but what affects them most is the trigger of various feelings that might have been from past experiences relating to the present ongoing circumstances.

The Past Oriented People

Past oriented people are people who dwell in the past. Their focus is often on the events of the past and most of the time you will find them being connected to past artifacts. These types of people are divided into two clusters. There might be the negated kind or the positive kind. The positive kind is often one that is accompanied by warm feelings. The past haunts these people in a way that gives them a positive sentiment. It could be from an event in the past or person in the past. These types of people are cohesive and are appreciative of how far they have come. The negated kind have the same negated approach towards life. Often these people are adhesive towards other people in life. They have connections in the past that make them look at life in a manner that suggests they are hurting. This spontaneous reaction is often exhibited in how they interact with people.

In order to achieve the positive psychology of time, there are some factors that need to be put into consideration. First, your overall outlook on time should change for the better. You have to balance your events on the time perspectives on the scale of balance. You do this by adopting a positive approach to life. With this type of mindset, you approach life in a more cynical manner in that you cannot dwell on the events of a particular day to be a determinant of what happens for the rest of your life. When you do this, it is said that you have achieved a balanced perspective on life. Balancing your perspectives about life will require that you focus all your attention on what makes you happy in life. This way you save your time more. You save your time more by being able to move on from traumatizing events rather than letting them take a toll on you. You are in control of your emotions and your body responds in a manner that suggests so. You are able to move from one task to another without undue waste of time. It is more often than not that you will find a person building castles in the air. This could be a result of an event that might have happened in the past. When this happens, you tend to waste a lot of time trying to shift back to your thoughts.

To understand how to use time wisely will require that we learn a few tricks on how to manipulate the little time we have. Normally the little time we have has very little effect on us when we put it into the right use. You may have probably attended a lecture on how best you can manage time. During this time, you are exposed to a number of tricks I which you can use in order to achieve maximum use of time as a resource. Research has it that despite this fact, people tend to throw in and go back to their previous behaviors.

When taking this utility of time, we ought to focus on a few pointers that will count a lot when it comes to utilization. Focusing on the wrong pointers, for instance, makes an individual waste a lot of the resource learning how to counter it in a way that will not happen. In order to achieve efficient use of time, we would first begin with motivation. In order to achieve efficiency in time management, you need to motivate yourself to focus on the things that will make you use time wisely. Normally these type of activities is not appealing to an individual. This is because they are strenuous in that they tend to curb the act of time-wasting. In order to achieve motivation, you need to focus your radar on the activities that are appealing to you. When you achieve this, you are able to engage in those activities without generating the feeling of monotony or boredom.

You ought to balance your schedule in order to fit your work and leisure correctly. You need not allocate so much time to leisure because your work is what pays the bills and gives you that luxurious lifestyle. You also ought not to forget leisure.

Leisure is what brings sense to all your hard work. Remember all work and no play makes John a dull boy.

Chapter 9: Negative Thinking

Destruction Of Negative Thinking Pattern

Have you heard about a simple method that is being used globally by subconscious awareness to destroy negative thinking patterns? It means that many people, just like you, have become more confident and have eliminated the concerns of others.

Thinking negatively can, in many ways affect your life. It can hold you back and make you feel wretched. A negative thought can easily be a bad habit, and we all know that bad habits are so difficult to break. You will feel miserable, sad, and worried if you continuously think negative thinking and believe what you are thinking.

The "true" you are going to be hidden.

Moreover, your subconscious mind automatically runs your entire body. It's your car pilot-your spacecraft. Anything in your subconscious will reflect the way you feel and act. Remember that you will destroy negative patterns of thinking by controlling how your subconscious works.

Therefore, if you say: I feel so self-conscious, I don't know I'm going to be so anxious to do it...

Then you will be a self-conscious, unconfident, anxious person.

Simple! Simple like that!

Furthermore, I want to tell you a true but unbelievable tale of a man who was thinking he was dead because he thought he was locked in a freight train freezer overnight. The reality is, yes, it was accidentally locked in the freezer compartment, but it wasn't turned on! However, he thought it was, and therefore his subconscious made his body react accordingly so that his heart eventually slowed down and stopped!

That's how powerful your mind can be-so watch out for what you think!

In addition, Promise yourself to become more aware of what thoughts your head enters. Stop thinking stuff like: I am the worst driver in the world. I'm going to mess up the series. There's no chance he/she would like to get out with me today. The catalyst that controls your subconscious destroys negative thinking patterns forever. Ask yourself whether a particular thought will be good or bad for you. Will it affect your life positively or negatively?

Analyze every thought: Are you indeed the world's worst driver?

Will it be so bad if this presentation is messed up? Is the world going to end?

How do you know he or she doesn't want to go out with you? That's what you think. So, you don't see the result, you can't read minds.

Controlling Negative Thinking

Negative thoughts could have significant and detrimental impacts on our lives. You must find ways to overcome negative thinking to make the most of life. We all have self-destroying, limited thoughts, at some point, when embarking upon a new goal, challenge, enterprise, or experience. For many, such negative thinking often leads to so many goals and dreams being abandoned.

When negative thinking takes hold, it gives you the chance to thrive, and to achieve success in the world. I succumbed so often in my life to this debilitating way of thinking that did not cause me an end to struggle, pain, and frustration. The fact is that success, prosperity, and happiness are rights granted to all of us. Nevertheless, the expectation that this is accomplished depends on the fact that all negative and minimal thoughts are eradicated from one's life.

Below, I want to recommend smooth but very successful ways to overcome negative thinking habits regularly:

1. **Smile:** This is the easiest way to deal with negative thoughts. It becomes harder to think negatively if you have a smile on your face. And it's contagious; it's going to make people smile around you. Ask yourself if you're in a bad mood and don't feel like smiling. You're going to feel better before you know it.

2. **Write. Sing:** Probably one of the best ways to overcome negative thinking is to play and sing joyfully. Although you don't know the lyrics, only the singing act can put you in a positive mood immediately.

3. **Remember the things for which you are grateful:**

It helps to remember the positive when the power of negative thoughts overcomes you. Sit down and list the things for which you are grateful. It can be just as easy as a sunny day, a repeat of a favorite TV show and good food, or as big as an unused medicine, advertisements, and answered prayer.

4. **A sense of humor. Have a sense of humor:**

If things don't go as you planned and you begin to feel bad, try to keep your humor right. Yes, it can be tough, but as soon as you learn how to see the funny side, mistakes and blunders will not hit you as much as they used to.

5. **Using Positive Affirmations:** Positive declarations are positive statements that you say to yourself or yourself again and again.

This not only will the overall mood be raised by repeating these positive affirmations with emotion and feeling, but it will also begin to question and remove deep-seated negative beliefs within your subconscious mind and introduce more optimistic and motivating ideas.

6. Get Active Research showed that exercise and physical activity promote the development of endorphins or "happy chemicals" in the brain that increase your mood and make you feel good. When I feel a bit nervous or frustrated, riding on a bicycle will always be great for my state of mind.

7. **Surround Yourself With Thinkers Positive.**

If you are caught in a loop of misery, it will not help to be around people who foster your negative thinking. Sometimes it's worth having friends that will help you put things into perspective and inspire you.

8. **Perform yoga and meditation — yoga training.**

These exercises teach you to be calm and help to achieve emotional and spiritual peace so that your thoughts and mind are more controlled.

9. **Think positive. Think positive.**

To overcome negative thinking, try shifting from negative to positive the tone of your thinking. Instead of saying, "This will be a challenging month for our group," reassure yourself, "This month, we are going to have some interesting challenges, but if we work together and do our utmost, all will be rewarding at last."

10. **Help Someone. Help Someone.**

Sometimes the best way to overcome negative thinking is to turn your attention back. Do something for someone else. Just simple acts of kindness and selflessness take things away from you and leave you with a feeling of happiness.

11. **Accept failure. Accept failure**

Another way of overcoming negative thoughts is to stop the fear of failure. Be comfortable. Be comfortable with it. Like it. Love it. Regardless of how much you try to avoid failure, accept it is part of life.

12.**Take your life responsibility.**

You've got options. When you feel stuck, realize that nobody can stop you from progressing and rising in your life. Don't play the victim. Don't play the victim. Be your own destiny's boss. This is one of the best ways to overcome negative thinking: know that you are creating your own life.

The effects of a negative attitude are a life of struggle and hotness. The way you think is the essential thing in life to attract and achieve. Discover a proven method to overcome negative thinking forever so that you finally can build an experience you have always dreamt of.

Dangerous Patterns to Avoid

Do you know that most of what makes us worried and anxious are just the byproducts of a poorly trained, full mind? There are ways to keep your head unclouded and positively. All you have to do is train and shape your mind, and the best way to do that is to program subliminally.

It involves sending messages to your subconscious so that they can work in a certain way and follow a particular direction towards the positive, not negative.

But to make the mindfully positive, you must look for some dangerous patterns of thought. These are common ways that the mind works; we sometimes lack control over them so that we can lead them to fear and undue concern. They are here:

1. **You're not a lucky man:** People get used to predicting what will happen to them each time they take action or decision. For example, you have just got a new job, and you start to imagine all the ways that your unique chance might be misled. We often hear ourselves saying, "I knew it was going to happen" or "I know it ends badly." This shows that we are wired to expect the worst results. The worst part is that the mind works to realize what it trusts, so what you hope will happen.

2. **Making assumptions:** Make assumptions. Here's another fickle habit: believing what others feel without hearing them say such things necessarily. It triggers a reaction in your head when you assume. And if what you felt was incorrect, your answer is also uninvited. This is often the first cause of trouble that could come first of all have been avoided.

Apart from this, perceptions create fear, doubts about oneself, low self-esteem, and degraded confidence.

3. **Making widespread** Another bad habit of avoiding is to make your negative experiences and actions generalized. This often happens when they label and mess things up incorrectly. We begin to think about how we never get right or how we

always make mistakes. Sometimes mistakes occur, but not always. They are easy to see, and concentrating on them, making it look bigger than it is, will only lead to anxiety and a negative self-image.

4. **Do not label yourself.** Do not label yourself. You will label yourself as the girl who always makes mistakes, or you will find yourself dumped. Why? Why? Because the mind works to realize its convictions. The mind cannot stand it if the truth is inconsistent with what it believes. It is, therefore, hard to keep the label you put on yourself.

5. **Out of anthills mountains**: Yes, you sometimes find problems that look like mountains and feel like you can't get out of it. But the bigger they get and the less capable you think of solving them if you continue to think of them as huge problems. This creates feelings of impotence and inferiority. Instead of thinking about your big problem, solve it.

Control of Anxiety and Negative Thinking

Everybody is involved. But if you get concerned about your work, your health, or your standard of living, you can develop an anxiety disorder. You may have physical symptoms, such as sleeplessness and headaches, which may make it harder for you to work in daily life if you have an anxiety disorder.

Sometimes everyone is nervous. Unfortunately, many people are always worried. Anxiety is part of our defense system against potential threats. Unfortunately, it becomes a condition when the depression becomes so bad that the patient is not able to cope.

There are a variety of types of anxiety disorders. The medical profession diagnoses them by specific types: Generalized anxiety disorder (GAD). The constant feeling of anxiety and concern characterizes this. Sometimes, there is no particular problem that causes concern. To be diagnosed with GAD, the extreme interest has to last for more than six months. Both men and women may develop this disorder (although more women tend to seek GAD help in statistical terms).

Furthermore, the disorder of social anxiety (social phobia). Individuals with social phobia are uncomfortable in social situations. This could range from critical events, like speaking publicly or speaking, to simple conditions like socializing with a few friends. We hate social situations because they are afraid of criticism and embarrassment. The disease is thought to be a genetic predisposition.

Obsessive-compulsive (OCD) disorder. People who suffer from OCD become concerned with certain thoughts and anxieties, such as wondering if the door is locked and fear of dust or germs. Obsessive habits, such as gate locking, locks re-checking, and frequent hand washing, relieve these anxieties.

In addition, panic disorder. Panic disorder. Individuals with panic disorder experience acute anxiety and extreme physical signs. A panic attack can lead you to think that you have a heart attack or that you will die. The panic attack's physical effects can include respiratory shortness, palpitation, tightness, dizziness, and sweat. There are no warnings or sources of assault. In women, panic disorder is more common than in men.

Post-traumatic stress disorder. Post-traumatic stress disorder. This disorder happens in people who have experienced violent or traumatic events. We often have retrofits to the case and can avoid people or circumstances in which their experience can be remembered. Sometimes they feel anxious and can be easily frightened or shocked.

Worry, anxiety, and stress are growing components of everyday life. But, when depression takes your life, you may need help to control it.

NLP has various techniques to help people overcome their anxiety problems. NLP targets behavior, words, and attitudes that hurt one's life and changes negative beliefs and produces positive results with simple techniques.

For example, the' swish pattern' is a common NLP technique. An NLP therapist works with a client to understand what causes depression, often a negative customer's self-image. NLP teaches how to replace a positive self-image of harmful anxiety.

One NLP stress approach is the use of anchoring. Anchoring is where a positive emotional state is created to replace a negative' anxious' state. This optimistic state is' anchored,' which means that a signal is generated to activate the state when the subject starts to feel fear-that anchor could be an accidental physical contact.

Self-Help Fitness Habit

Let's start with the evidence. We must all exercise. Some of us are doing that already; others are doing a little bit; most of us might be using more. It's not a surprise, and it's not one of those kinds of things where "maybe this could help." It is a scientifically proven fact that everyone can benefit from incorporating exercise into their lifestyles in terms of health, quality of life, and longevity. It's an argument of fitness that's open and shut.

As noted, though, millions of us do not exercise and millions more who do not exercise enough. It seems like an insane bit of stupidity. Here's something we know our lives will change in every way, but we don't do it yet. We find ways to spend our time doing things that are far less productive every day, but so many of us don't practice the way we should.

Well, that's irrational. That does not say, however, that it is incomprehensible. You see, we're just habit creatures. This is a natural tendency for human beings. The practice is work. It can be fun, it's gratifying, but it takes effort. Human beings seem to be hardwired whenever possible to avoid unnecessary exertion (a potential remnant of our evolution).

So, naturally, if we don't have to do that, we don't want to exercise, and we can quickly form the habits. That's why we don't work out the way we ought to.

The exercise needs to be recognized by our intellects. But the skin is not budding. What's the answer? In view of all the potential gains from a healthier lifestyle, surrender does not make much sense, so it leaves on the alternative: self-help.

Sure, eventually, each of us should decide to exercise more and take the necessary steps to turn that decision into a physical reality. This will require some self-help in changing our current bad habits and overcoming the natural tendency not to break a sweat if we don't have to. Fortunately, there are plenty of great self-help resources that can get a body off the couch and into practice.

Starting with small things is a great way to begin your self-help exercise by incorporating a little extra physical activity into your daily life. You know the drill, you know... Take the stars, give the pet a walk— or perhaps walk around the block holding your spouse's hands and talking about the day. While you're going, it doesn't matter.

A great way to break a habit is to be attracted to a more attractive alternative. The simple notion of self-help suggests that if you choose things you enjoy, you'll have more luck getting yourself to exercise regularly. Make it amusing, not grinding.

Don't bite as much as you can chew. Sure, you want to set yourself high goals and work towards them. Though, in trying to reach the larger goals too fast or on an arbitrary timeline, you don't want to undermine such self-help initiatives. Divide your exercise goals into manageable single hunks that you can deal with more quickly.

Track the progress you have made. Any self-help specialist would inform you that it is much easier to do away with bad behaviors when you start to see positive results. Keep a log for the workout. Keep track of your achievements along the way. Find a way to remember how you're making progress. The very production of these reminders will assist you in the development of winning training habits.

They can't deny the fitness advantages, so why don't so many of us do what we should do? The answer is straightforward. We've got bad habits that are difficult to beat. Thankfully, a little effort and some validated self-help techniques will help us to conquer these negative behaviors, helping us to finally enjoy some of the obvious benefits of adding more physical activity to our lives!

Active Exercise for Self-Help

Many forms of self-help are being used. Such approaches are designed to make a happier and more successful life for you. Self-help is increasingly focused on curbing various areas of life, such as diseases and unproductive lives. Here are five methods for self-help, which can change your life.

Method 1: Affirmations These are simple and straightforward affirmative statements indicating either your current positive status or decisive action. Affirmations must be repeated many times to affect the subconscious mind. As the subconscious mind begins to believe the claims are valid, it helps you align your thoughts with your actions. It, in effect, helps to bring you closer to your dream life.

Daily statements include statements such as, "I'm beautiful," "I'm going to succeed in this mission," "I'm unique and special," and "Losing that job will only lead me to a better job."

Method 2: Target setting This is an excellent method for self-help. By having a plan, it's hard to plan to succeed. Hence, make every effort to achieve them after setting goals. This will boost your self-esteem and increase your chances of further success significantly.

Method 3: Creative Visualizations This is an excellent self-help tool. To do this, imagine the success of anything you want to do. Doing this on an ongoing basis will help you begin to believe it as accurate. This will increase your chances of this occurring dramatically.

Method 4: Meditation is a highly effective method for self-help. This is a technique in which a person trains his mind to trigger a particular mode of consciousness to gain an expected advantage. Meditation has many benefits. Some of them are outlined below: it reduces cortisol production; the stress hormone It boosts the immune system It reduces chronic pain It increases longevity It reduces high blood pressure The fact that meditation is suitable for both your mind and your body. The subconscious mind is actively trying to communicate with your conscious mind. This message will be delivered through your body if you don't pay attention. This may be due to body pains, diseases, cramps, muscle tension, and many other body dysfunctions. To avoid all this, meditation helps.

Method 5: Exercise is one thing that most people know about, but very few people do. You don't have to go to a clinic to start exercising unless you have a unique condition. The first step you should take towards fitness is to increase your activity level. Monitor any patterns that will stop you from sitting down and make you more involved depending on machines.

Conclusively, it's not enough to increase your level of activity alone. It is essential to create and adhere to a particular exercise routine. Just change for the better if you need to change your method. You don't have to go to the gym automatically. You can go for aerobics, jogging, running, taking a brisk walk, swimming vigorously and regularly, dancing or playing an active sport. A better mood for better health Increased energy Having a better physique Keeping weight in check. The first step to self-help is to decide to take control of your life. Stop letting it affect other people. Stop assuming things are going to be all right in the future. Instead, to ensure a brighter future, start using these self-help techniques now.

Tips for Self-Help Confidence

Imagine being able to take life head-on by embracing the way you are and learning to be a better person from past mistakes. What must you do? You and you alone can change your view of yourself and how others look at you. This can be achieved by using trusting techniques of self-help to bring your level of trust to the best it can be.

What are some methods of self-help confidence that you can use to improve yourself?

You need to ask yourself this question, "What is it that I want to change about me?" After you come up with a list of things you need to change, then it's time to look at the different ways you can accomplish this. Let's try them out, are we going to?

Experiment with something different. Carrying out a challenging task that meets your limits will help you identify skills you have never learned. This will allow you to break through personal barriers that you have built to reach to higher levels of your limitations.

Make plans that you can achieve. You may have performed tasks before, but you fell on the way due to a lack of confidence. Every time it's going to be different because you've got to set realistic targets, you've got to see through. This will tell you that you can do more than you do at the moment.

Moreso, read materials to motivate you. There are different sources online as well as in bookstores that have stories written by people who have experienced the same as the one you are experiencing. Once you know that you're not the only one that's going through this thing, you're going to get inspired to get rid of your trust issues.

Regular Exercise: Moderate physical activity will increase your level of energy and ensure that you are in a positive state. During exercise, the positivity comes from releasing endorphins and testosterone in the body. Exercise helps you get in shape and enhance your appearance to make you feel more comfortable.

Overcome the anxieties. Most of the time, there is a lack of confidence due to fear that has grown in you and has become chronic. Make sure this is not an easy task, and you need to be prepared mentally. Slowly take the necessary steps to embrace the fear. Find different ways to approach this fear and try to find the most effective.

Eliminate negative memories, accept those that are good. Do not allow your mind to be enveloped by previous bad experiences and mistakes until you solve an important issue. Try to counter this as much as you can by thinking about positive achievements, skills, and memories that will help you focus better on the task ahead.

Therefore, no matter what people say about you, you shouldn't take it on your own. Take your time to enjoy yourself. Through recognizing your strengths and working on getting them out, while suppressing your negative traits, you can do this.

In addition, enhance your social skills. Friends and colleagues are a vital component to lift the level of trust. Learn how to speak and interact with people, these self-help techniques will go a long way to enhance your trust and help you live a happy, relaxed life.

Conclusion

I will first commence by extending my greatest gratitude to you the readers for making it this far. Most people tend to give up on the way. This book has taken you through many episodes and I will only seek to give you a recap. In the first chapter, you got to know what psychology is. The initial chapter went ahead to highlight the in-depth of psychology stating its tenets. We discussed the aspects that psychology seeks to meet and saw it was only to give you some examples in an attempt to elaborate further. The chapter comes to an end with a focus on the perspectives of psychology. This gave you an overview of what psychology entails.

Shifting our focus to chapter two, we go to comprehend how to use psychology to our advantage. With the few tricks elaborated we had a feel of how it was when we analyzed people using the psychology at hand. The four tenets of psychology highlighted here were: behavioral psychology, psychodynamic approach cognitive psychology and not forgetting biological approach. Chapter three presents the fields in which psychology can be applied. The emerging trends in psychology have been outlined here and each has been elaborated alongside its relevance.

Chapter four exposes psychology at a personal level. At this level, we get to know about the various challenges that an individual faces. This includes the various disorders that come as a result. The disorders include personality disorders, dissociative disorders, mood disorders, stress depression and anxiety taking the helm. The art of social psychology is also mentioned and elaborated at this level. Chapter 5 brings about the methodology. This focuses on Darwin's theory of evolution. The chapter also explains why evolution is key. The chapter closes by discussing the evolution that is taking place today.

Chapter six comes in in a bid to explain how psychology functions. The structure of psychology is discussed keenly against the physiology behind psychology. The nervous system together with the endocrine system is discussed in lengths. The chapter then closes there. Chapter seven is a basic guideline that is in a bid to aid individuals who seek to further apply psychology. The chapter elaborates on various issues not limited to mindset, what is the right mindset when engaging in psychology? It goes further to include the active mind, motivation, and goal as subtopics. Nutrition optimism and physical exercise are not left out in this venture. Optimism is always key when it comes to taming the mind.

The chapter is keen to discuss the positive psychology of time. This chapter attempts to combine the two complex topics of psychology and time. Here the reader is exposed to various ways in which their positive psychology can be of aid when conserving time. The reader gets to know about the perspective of time and the various tenses involved. The chapter concludes by showing the reader how best to conserve time.

Finally, I wish to thank the reader for reading this book. There are many books but you chose this one.

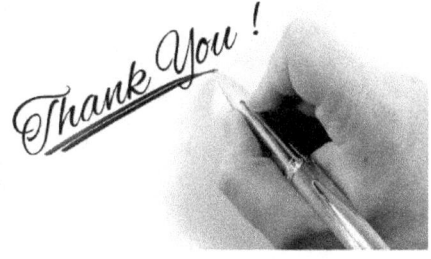

DR. Felicity Gray